Groupwork in Occupational Therapy

Groupwork in Occupational Therapy

Linda Finlay
Occupational Therapy Consultant
York
UK

Consultant Editor
Jo Campling

First published in 1993 by Chapman & Hall
Reprinted in 1997 by Stanley Thornes (Publishers) Ltd

Reprinted in 2001 by:
Nelson Thornes Ltd
Delta Place
27 Bath Road
CHELTENHAM
GL53 7TH
United Kingdom

05 06 / 12 11 10 9 8

A catalogue record for this book is available from the British Library

ISBN 0 7487 3636 0

Typeset by Best-set

Printed and bound in Spain by GraphyCems

Contents

Preface

There are many books available on groups and groupwork but few address the unique needs and approaches of occupational therapists. Current literature tends to focus on particular groups – psychotherapy for instance – and whilst they may be good in their own right they are designed for the needs of other disciplines. Occupational therapists need a groupwork text that selectively encompasses the theory of group dynamics and applies it to our specific range of groups.

This book applies general group theory to occupational therapy practice and aims to help therapists function more effectively in groups – be it as a leader or as a group member. I have tried to explore the full range of occupational therapy groupwork, from groups which emphasize our activity base and the development of skills, through to psychotherapy groups which stress dealing with emotions. Over and above the use of groups in therapy, all occupational therapists have to operate within staff groups and multi-disciplinary teams where the theory of groupwork can also be applied.

Therapists, students, support staff and tutors who are faced with the task of running a group – be it a cookery group, psychodrama, staff meeting or seminar – should all find this text useful. It is geared primarily to therapists working in the psycho-social field (both mental health and for people with learning difficulties), but I hope therapists in the physical and educational field will also find it helpful.

The book is divided into two parts. Part One tackles the theory of groupwork and focuses on how to understand groups and group processes. Part Two has a more practical bias and focuses on how to manage a group from the initial planning stage through to running and evaluating the group. The reader may either read the book sequentially or go straight to the subject of particular concern.

Chapter 1 offers an overview of the range and scope of groupwork in occupational therapy. Chapters 2 and 3 indicate some theoretical foundations for such work and more particularly explore the aspects of group dynamics which underlie all groups. Chapters 4 and 5 detail the practical considerations involved in planning groups, and offer guidelines for the preparation of one-off sessions and setting up longer term groups. Chapter 6 focuses specifically on leadership. It discusses the roles and styles we can adopt as leaders and the issues involved with co-leadership. Chapter 7 explores some problems which occur in groups and how as leaders we might manage them. Chapter 8 examines the importance of evaluation at all levels from recording groups to research. Chapter 9 concludes by outlining ways to develop group experience and group leader skills.

Throughout this book, I have sought to emphasize the practical application of groupwork in occupational therapy. Each chapter contains many case studies and practical examples. In addition, I have provided illustrative theory into practice boxes which highlight 'how to do' aspects of the matter under discussion.

The case examples offered relate to a variety of different types of groups, leaders and settings. Whilst most of the examples refer to patients and clients, others are drawn from staff and student groups. Both the physical and psycho-social fields of occupational therapy encompassed apply to hospital, community and educational settings.

Throughout the book I have sought to convey the importance of 'understanding'. An effective group therapist needs to understand the individuals who make up the group as well as people and the dynamics of their combined behaviour. Such understanding requires a balance of both analysis and empathy. On the **analysis** side, we must be able to stand back from the group and reflect on group processes. We need to plan our groups systematically and be clear (even deliberate) about the best way to ensure that our practice is therapeutic. We also have to evaluate the group and work out problems as they arise. Intellectual understanding is not enough, however. A group leader also needs **empathy**. We need to be aware of the strange, powerful emotions and motivations that a group can evoke. In addition, we have to be aware of, and use, our own feelings as a member of the group we are running. In this context, it helps if we can take opportunities to be a group member in other groups – to experience both the stress and the sharing which as a leader we will need to control. Achieving a balance of these two levels of understanding is one important challenge we face as therapists.

Having outlined what this book is intended to do, I would like also to mention its limits. I have restricted its scope to how to use elements of a group in a therapeutic way. I have not engaged in the debate about the merits of group therapy over individual work. I neither discuss who best benefits from groups nor offer judgements about who is best qualified to lead a group. These are professional decisions that need to be made jointly with our patients and clients and within the context of the treatment team and setting. The book will not turn a novice groupworker into an expert. It does demonstrate how to analyse group processes and offers ideas for practice, but this is only the first step. No amount of book learning can replace actual experience, both of being in, and of leading, groups.

In conclusion, I would like to acknowledge a number of people who contributed to the development of this book. I wish to thank the staff of Roundhay Wing, St James's University Hospital who helped me to explore issues and ideas about groupwork in practice. I am grateful to all the staff and students of the University College of Ripon and York St John who continue to encourage and support my efforts. My particular thanks go to Rick Telford, Chris Mayers and Robert Looker, all of whom offered their time and invaluable constructive advice on my first draft. I also wish to express special thanks to Malcolm Wilder for his continuing and immeasurable help and support. Finally, my gratitude needs to be given to both my editor Jo Campling and to Terri Cooper, editor of Chapman and Hall for their patience and helpful comments on the completed draft. In the last analysis, I alone remain responsible for any errors of content that may be found in the following pages. This book is dedicated to all the people who have taken part in the groups I have run – you have given meaning to my work.

Glossary

Activity group – Activity groups aim to develop skills and/or encourage social interaction. The term is used in contrast to 'support group' which emphasizes communication and psychotherapy elements.

Adapting (treatment) – Process by which treatment activities are modified to suit the background, ability and values of individuals or the circumstances of the situation.

Brain-storming – Spontaneous discussion technique used for generating ideas and creative thinking. Words and thoughts triggered in association with a particular topic are listed without initial evaluation.

Cohesion – Group process which occurs when members feel close or connected to each other and have a sense of belonging to a valued group.

Consensual validation – Interpersonal feedback offered by others which allows comparison with one's own self-evaluations. The process helps people develop a self-concept based on the appraisals of significant others.

Counter-transference – An unconscious process where a person responds to anothers transference with a further transference in return.

Directive group – Structured activity group designed by Kaplan (1984), based on the model of human occupation, for lower functioning psychiatric patients or clients who have performance difficulties.

Functional group – Activity group designed by Howe and Swartzberg (1984) to enhance the occupational behaviour of participants.

Grading (treatment) – A process by which the demands of an activity and/or the environment are progressively increased or decreased.

Group dynamics – The forces, social structures, behaviours, relationships and processes which occur within groups.

Group polarization – Process which can occur during group decision-making where members become more extreme in their opinions or stance.

Group think – Phenomenon where members in highly cohesive decision-making groups strive for unanimity. Critical evaluation of ideas takes second place to consensus.

Norms – Standard, customary ways of behaving in a group.

Optimal arousal level – Level at which group members feel energized and alert whilst feeling a little anxious and so challenged.

Process illumination – Technique employed in psychotherapy where the underlying dynamics of the group are brought into focus. Inter-group relationships and processes which are occuring at the time are explained.

Projective art – The medium of art is used as a psychodynamic technique to encourage the exploration of feelings. Feelings are 'projected' onto paper (or some other art medium).

Project group – Structured group designed by Mosey (1973) which aims to facilitate the development of group interaction skills appropriate to the group level. The project group aims to encourage basic sharing and interaction.

Psychodrama – The dramatic therapy technique devised by Moreno where individuals enact life scenes in order to explore their emotions, relationships and unconscious needs.

Risky-shift – An example of group polarization where group discussion results in higher risk choices compared to the choices individuals have made previously.

Social skills training – A behavioural technique designed to teach, systematically, elements of social behaviour using role-play, modelling and feedback.

Sociogram – (also called sociometric test) An analytical tool developed by Moreno (1953) to give insight into the underlying social structure of a group. The inter-relationships of group members are diagrammatically represented.

Support group – Support groups aim to help members to explore their feelings and give each other support. The term is used in contrast to 'activity group' which emphasizes task or social elements.

Transference – An unconscious process where a person responds to another in a manner similar to the way he or she responded to a significant person in the past, i.e. feelings are 'transferred'.

Part One

Understanding groups

1

Groups in occupational therapy

GROUPS IN SOCIETY

What we mean by 'society' is in large part the activity of people in groups of one kind or another. As we grow, work or simply live in society each one of us participates in a multitude of groups. We are born into a family group. At school we have classroom groups, sport groups, gossip groups, and at work there are team meetings, cooperative work tasks and informal discussions. In our social life we join clubs and societies, we meet with friends and 'do things' together. In all of these examples the group is more than just a collection of individuals. The members are bonded together both by their group identity and shared purposes which will only be achieved by interacting and working together (Mosey, 1973). Each group is unique. Some groups are relatively constant (such as the family), others continuously reform (like social groups). Some involve highly formal and structured activities, whilst others are informal and may involve us in simply being with others in a companionable silence.

Our social development is powerfully shaped by our experience of groups. We learn who we are as we interact with others. Our sense of identity comes from being in groups, for we adopt certain roles and respond to the expectations of other people. Arguably our very survival depends on our being able to cooperate with others in group tasks. Groups are more than a collection of individuals. As Blair says, groups are 'intrinsic to our existence' (1990, p 194).

The therapeutic group is one special kind of group. This chapter explains the particular characteristics of groups which cause them to be a valuable vehicle for therapy and then shows how occupational therapists select different types of group activity to expose patients and clients to the learning experience they seek.

GROUPS IN THERAPY

In order to be able to examine the role of groups in therapy, we must first identify some of the key features of groups which therapists will seek to tap into and use. Groups are a natural learning environment, and within a group many complex interactions occur. Every individual in the group communicates with every other individual in the group at all times. This means that there are **multiple layers of relationships** within the group developing and changing moment by moment, and members can draw on the therapeutic potential of having relationships with several people at once rather than working with just one therapist. Groups involve **sharing and support**. Within them we share others' pains, pleasures and accomplishments. We gain strength from feeling connected to others and having others accept us. Groups are a dynamic **source of energy** and creativity. When people in a group are actively bouncing ideas off of each other the experience is stimulating. Groups provide the opportunity for **social learning** as we interact, model on and advise each other. The experience of being in a group can **heighten emotions** helping them to be expressed and explored. Emotions spread and amplify in a group in a way that is contagious. Finally, groups are powerful shapers of behaviour (positively and negatively) as group **norms and pressure** ensure that we respond to others' expectations and demands upon us.

These special qualities of groups, summarized in Figure 1.1, are the qualities we try to harness for use within therapy.

Curative factors

The theoretical rationale for all group therapy is founded on the curative dynamics of group activity. However this may be expressed, used or understood, the dynamics of interdependent people relating to each other in groups is endlessly challenging. Our success as group therapists depends entirely upon our

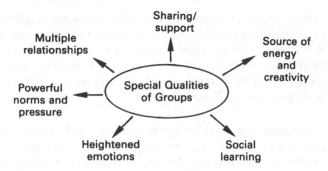

Figure 1.1 Summary of special qualities of groups.

capacity to unfold and sensitively manage these complex events.

The foundation of current practice in group therapy and the touchstone for much research is Yalom's 11 curative factors of group therapy (Yalom, 1975). Yalom's conclusions about the value of group therapy are briefly summarized below.

1. *Instillation of hope.* A patient or client needs hope to keep in treatment, and faith that treatment can be therapeutic in itself. The therapist must believe in the positive benefits of the group and convey them to the group members if it is to stand a chance of success. Groups such as Alcoholics Anonymous are said to work effectively, precisely because the members act as inspiration for each other.

2. *Universality.* As group members share their experiences they come to understand they are not alone and their problems are not unique. They find it enormously therapeutic to have the opportunity to disclose (perhaps previously hidden) feelings to a group of people who are willing to listen, and not judge.

3. *Imparting information.* Groups provide a key learning forum for their members. Such learning may be formal through lectures, demonstrations or films, or more informal as members gain from giving each other advice or suggestions.

4. *Altruism.* Yalom emphasizes that group members gain from the 'intrinsic act of giving' (Yalom, 1974, p 13). They can offer

each other support, reassurance, suggestions, insight and sharing of similar problems. Often patients or clients will listen and absorb observations from another member far more readily than from the therapist. The fact that group members can be of importance to others can be of particular value in boosting their self-confidence and self-esteem.

5. *The corrective recapitulation of the primary family group.* Group processes can simulate the family group by allowing patients and clients to work through family problems. For example, if a group has a male and a female therapist they may represent the parental roles while the other group members become siblings. Members may project their feelings onto others, exploring old feelings and experimenting with new interactions.

6. *Development of socializing techniques.* Social learning and the development of basic social skills occurs in all groups. Patients and clients can learn and practise social skills through role-play or games which can then be reinforced by giving each other feedback about how they come across.

7. *Imitative behaviour.* Group members can model on each other and on the therapist and learn new ways of behaving. Members may also benefit vicariously by observing the therapy of another person.

8. *Interpersonal learning.* The group is a social microcosm where behaviours from a person's normal social environment are demonstrated in the group and behaviour learned in the group is carried through outside. As humans we need to interact with others and gain their acceptance. Mental illness can result when normal relationships are disturbed. People need 'consensual validation' from others which enables them to view themselves differently. A group can also help members to self-reflect on their emotions, behaviour and relationships. Learning occurs throughout all of these processes.

9. *Group cohesiveness.* Yalom makes an analogy between cohesiveness in group therapy and the 'relationship' in individual therapy. Cohesiveness is a significant curative factor because in conditions of acceptance patients and clients are

more inclined to express themselves and hence become more self-aware. Research demonstrates that cohesive groups more powerfully shape social behaviour, increase self-esteem, are more stable, and have better attendance (a vital element in successful therapy) compared to non-cohesive groups.

10. *Catharsis.* Catharsis refers to the free expression of feelings. The value of catharsis is seen as a part of wider processes of cohesiveness, sharing and developing bonds. In therapy groups, members may benefit from learning how to express feelings or they may simply gain relief from 'getting things off their chest'.

11. *Existential factors.* Being part of a group allows the opportunity to come to terms with issues to do with 'responsibility, basic isolation, contingency, the recognition of our mortality . . . and the capriciousness of existence' (1974, p 85). Yalom notes that patients and clients often express important philosophical sentiments about the value of groups such as, 'recognising that no matter how close I get to other people, I still face life alone' (1974, p 84).

The full implications of these 11 curative factors cannot be absorbed quickly, but it is clear that groups are multi-layered, complex and powerful.

GROUPS IN OCCUPATIONAL THERAPY

Occupational therapists can use a variety of group situations to exploit the curative opportunities which groups offer. We try to identify the needs of our patients or clients and then seek an appropriate learning environment for them. This often means selecting a specific group experience. However, the curative benefits of group activity are neither random nor inevitable. The power of group events can be destructive as well as beneficial and therapists must learn to support patients and clients both in their selection of the group, and in their group learning experience.

Occupational therapists use a particularly wide range of groups, each with its own therapeutic function and purpose. I find it helpful to classify these groups into four types along a continuum. Figure 1.2 represents this continuum and shows

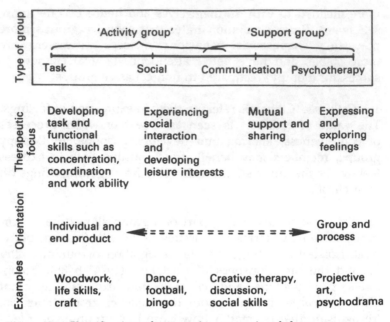

Figure 1.2 Classification of groups in occupational therapy.

the therapeutic aim and group orientation of each type of group. Examples of groups are indicated under each heading for illustration.

Groups can be distinguished in terms of whether they are predominantly activity-based, support-based, or a mixture of the two. Groups may therefore be classified according to their position on an activity–support continuum on which the main elements are **task, social, communication** and **psychotherapy**. This classification is based loosely on the work of DeMare and Kreegar (1974), who propose that groups can operate at three levels: psychotherapeutic, communicational and recreational.

'Activity groups' primarily involve task and/or social elements. **Task** groups aim to develop skills and tend to be end-product and individually orientated. Typical examples of task groups are work groups, craft groups, reality orientation, life skills groups etc. **Social** groups are for recreation and fun, and aim to encourage social interaction. Typical examples here are: music and movement, football, bingo and a newspaper group.

'Support groups' emphasize communication and psycho-therapy elements. In contrast to activity groups, support groups are group rather than individually orientated and their focus is on the group process more than the end product. **Communication** groups aim for group members to share experiences and give each other support. Some typical examples here are: a women's discussion group, music therapy, social skills training and art therapy. **Psychotherapy** groups aim to increase insight into individual's problems and help them to explore their feelings. Typical examples include: projective art, verbal psychotherapy, play therapy and psychodrama.

THEORY INTO PRACTICE

'Activity groups - task and social elements

Task group: (focus is on the activity or piece of work to be completed)

Typical aims	Example group	Typical goals
To develop task performance skills	Pottery group	sustain concentration for 45 min complete one coil pot adequately
To develop group interaction skills	Craft group	share tools and equipment appropriately initiate conversation with one person

Social group: (focus of activity is on enjoyment and fun)

Typical aims	Example group	Some example goals
To encourage social interaction	Dance group	ask at least one person to dance show awareness of non-verbal aspects such as touch, body space etc.

| To develop leisure pursuits | Sports group | learn a cooperative game
gain awareness of how a community facility may be used for leisure |

THEORY INTO PRACTICE

'*Support groups*' – communication and psychotherapy elements

Communication group: (emphasis is on sharing, caring and support)

Typical aims	Example group	Some example goals
To share experiences	Women's group	understand the difference between assertion, aggression and passivity disclose one relevant problem
To be sensitive to others' experiences	Music appreciation	quietly listen to the music discuss the different feelings evoked in members by the music

Psychotherapy group: (focus on feelings and interpersonal reactions)

Typical aims	Example group	Some example goals
To explore (or act out a problem situation	Psychodrama	It is inappropriate to set goals but individuals may set
Reduce sense of powerlessness and isolation through group identity	Verbal psychotherapy	their own such as 'to volunteer to act out own scenario within two sessions'

There are three further points relevant to my classification of groups which are worth noting here. First, any activity can be used in a variety of ways to meet different aims. Art, for example, can be applied either as a work task to build concentration or as a confidence boosting leisure activity. It can be used within art therapy and also in more analytically orientated projective art.

Second, any group activity can span several categories at once. A 'retirement group' is a good example where all the elements are on offer but these shift according to the exercise at hand and on different group members' responses. Thus members might simultaneously share feelings (psychotherapy), give each other support (communication), have fun (social) and develop skills in a new hobby (task).

Thirdly, different individuals may react differently to the same activity. A social skills training role-play, for instance, may be experienced by different individuals as a deeply emotional experience, as fun, or as simply hard work!

DIFFERENT APPROACHES TO GROUP WORK

So far, we have moved from a discussion of groups in society and the use of groups in therapy to a consideration of types of groups in occupational therapy. In this final section of Chapter 1, I would like to be even more specific about different types of approaches to groupwork. The examples discussed have the virtue of being well documented and backed by research. Collectively, they serve to demonstrate the enormous range and variety of uses to which groupwork in occupational therapy can be put. (For convenience, I have classified them in terms of the activity group/support group distinction spelt out in the previous section – see Table 1.1.)

Table 1.1 A selection of groups based on theory and research

Activity groups	Support groups
Developmental	Psychodrama
Directive group	Social skills training
Functional group	Psychodynamic communication group
Cognitive dysfunction	Creative therapy

Table 1.2 Summary of Mosey's group interaction skills

18 mths–2 years	Parallel group	able to work alongside others
2–4 years	Project group	minimally shares, competes, co-operates with therapist prompting
5–7 years	Egocentric-co-operative group	co-operates and competes, experiments with group roles
9–12 years	Co-operative group	meets needs of other members and expresses feelings
15–18 years	Mature group	flexibly takes on various roles

Developmental groups

The first of the activity groups I wish to describe is based on Anne Cronin Mosey's (1986) theory of adaptive skills which lays out six areas of functioning or 'adaptive skills'. These are further sub-divided into sequential sub-skills which can be used as treatment goals. The development of **group interaction skills** is particularly relevant to occupational therapy group-work. Patients or clients are placed into the 'group environment' (which includes the activity, therapist and other members) that best suits their developmental level. They are then encouraged to progress through the teaching–learning process. Table 1.2 above summarizes the basic stages.

Directive group

A second kind of activity group is proposed by Kathy Kaplan (1986), who has devised a specific, highly structured group based on the **model of human occupation** (Kielhofner, 1985) which she has named 'directive group'. The group is designed for lower functioning psychiatric patients who have perform-ance difficulties, namely in task performance, self care and basic interaction. Kaplan lays down the basic structure of the group – for instance that it meets daily and follows a set format. Two group leaders are directive and encourage members to take part in a range of group activities (such as crafts, games, exercises) relevant to the individual's and group's treatment goals.

Functional group

A third activity group to be considered is the Functional Group. The Functional Group, based on Howe and Swartzberg's (1986) 'groupwork model', aims to enhance the occupational behaviour of participants. Basic goals are to elicit purposeful, self-initiated, spontaneous and group-centred action in members who are required to make choices and to perform work, play and self-maintenance tasks. The leader uses five guidelines in seeking to influence the group process: 1) facilitate maximum **involvement through group-centred action** (for instance, by fully explaining the task to the members); 2) achieve maximum **sense of individual and group identity** through assigning individuals roles and creating a safe, stable group; 3) prompt **flow experience** by pleasurable activities; 4) facilitate **spontaneous involvement of members** by modelling and accepting behaviour; 5) encourage member **support and feedback**.

Cognitive dysfunction group

A final activity group is provided by Claudia Allen (1985) in her cognitive disabilities model. She delineates **six levels of cognitive function** (level 1 = client is conscious, reflexes are working but awareness and concentration are severely impaired; level 6 = client is normal, can plan actions and use symbolic cues). Patients or clients are placed in treatment activities which match their cognitive level. Earhart (1985) describes nine occupational therapy groups which can be used to treat the six levels of dysfunction. The groups are wide ranging, for instance, simple movement (level 2), crafts (level 3), work evaluation (level 6). Guidelines are provided for the therapist concerning the activity, method of instruction, equipment needed and the environment.

Psychodrama

Turning to support groups, one key example comes from Moreno, who established the technique of psychodrama – the 'theatre of spontaneity' (Moreno, 1946). Psychodrama combines psychotherapy, creative therapy and drama, and involves a person acting out and working through personal problems by re-creating difficult life events. The components of psychodrama are: 1) The **stage** where life dramas are re-enacted; 2) the **protagonist** who is the centre of the drama; 3) the **director** (therapist) who guides the drama; 4) the **auxiliary egos** who are the group members who act out the protagonist's characters; 5) the **audience** who take an active part by reacting and giving feedback. This intense therapy method can be seen as the forerunner to role play and behavioural rehearsal techniques which are widely used in therapy today.

Social skills training

A second type of support group is the behavioural technique of social skills training, which is designed to teach, systematically, elements of social behaviour (verbal, non-verbal, assertion etc.) to people. The techniques used include **role-play** or behavioural rehearsal, **modelling** and positive **feedback**. Franklin (1990) identifies four principles of skills training, namely: demonstration, guidance, practice and feedback. There are many models and approaches to social skills training. Argyle's work is perhaps the best known (see Argyle 1987 for an updated version).

Psychodynamic communication group

I use the title of 'psychodynamic communication group' to capture the essence of a type of support group devised by Gail and Jay Fidler (1963). They explore the psychodynamic aspects of occupational therapy in their emphasis of the unconscious, object relations and the symbolic potential of activities. They describe communication as the core of occupational therapy, specifically, how activities can help individuals to communicate thoughts and feelings. Interpersonal relations are seen as central and interactions in a group offer opportunities for sharing, ego-strengthening and reality testing. They describe how a group might be used to help members develop social awareness, cooperation and a sense of belonging to the group.

Creative therapy

The final example of a support group involves the application of the creative therapies. Art, drama, pottery, music, poetry are all **creative activities** which have been used in a psycho-therapeutic way to help individuals to gain insight into their inner conflicts and explore their feelings. Whilst creative therapy is an umbrella term rather than a specific type of group, I wanted to indicate that we can use the full range of such activities in occupational therapy. Creative therapy groupwork is advocated by theorists of both psycho-analytical and humanistic approaches, both of which will be considered in turn.

The early work of the Azimas (Azima, Cramer-Azima and Wittkower 1957) is a good example of the use of unstructured creative occupational therapy activities based on **psychoanalytic** principles. They propose that groups participate in free creative and association activities using art (namely pencil and paper, crayons or plasticine activities). The group's objectives are to work through defences, drives, transferences and conflicts, and help individuals to gain insight. The created object is used as an 'essential catalyst' in the group process (1959). For a fuller account of occupational therapy and group psychotherapy see Blair (1990).

A **humanistic** approach to creative therapy is suggested by gestalt principles and the work of Fredrick Perls (1974). Perls emphasizes the whole nature of a person's experience and here-and-now expressions where individuals are taught to describe rather than analyse feelings. Gestalt therapists often use sensory awareness or sensitivity exercises and drama encounters to help an individual become more self-aware.

This introductory chapter has explored the value and potential of groups in general. Then, more specifically, the broad range of groups which operate within occupational therapy have been described. Throughout the rest of the book, I shall give examples of this full range of therapeutic groups and use the classification offered. I hope to show how we can harness the special qualities of groups in our therapy practice.

2

Group dynamics: group processes

Underlying the apparent behaviour of a group, there is a rich tapestry of needs, motivations, interconnecting relationships and feelings about the group itself. Every group is unique and evolves in its own special way – depending on the individual members, the situation, and the events which occur in the group itself. The study of these processes concerning the nature of groups, how they develop and how they work, is called **group dynamics**.

Chapters 2 and 3 are about group dynamics. This chapter explores a range of processes which occur within groups. We examine the **roles** people play in groups, **relationships** between members, **interaction, non-verbal communication** and **decision-making.** The next chapter examines the specific process of how a group evolves through key **phases** over time. Both chapters first discuss the theory underpinning group dynamics (section A), then case examples are offered to illustrate how the theory can be used in practice (section B). Underlying this system of organization is my conviction that a grasp of the theoretical assumptions involved is a valuable aid to helping us understand the purpose and logic of groupwork. However, I also appreciate that many of us are less enthusiastic about 'theory' as such. Those of you who prefer to gloss over straight theory may find it easier to start with the latter sections, which provide practical examples of groups in action. You might then consider going back to the underlying theory to see whether, in practice, it helps to improve your grasp of group dynamics.

A. Group processes

ROLES

Roles people play in groups

Roles are social positions. In social situations people adopt certain attitudes and behaviours according to their own and others' expectations about how they should behave. I like Merton's (1957) definition of role as, '. . . the behavioural enacting of the patterned expectations attributed to a stated position.'

Group roles can be formally ascribed or informally adopted. The former involve an official position with its associated status and responsibilities. Examples of such roles are the occupational therapist, patient, head of department, helper, consultant, instructor, volunteer and student. People who have these positions will behave in the appointed role when they are in related groups.

In addition to their official roles, group members are likely to take on any of a range of informal roles. Some roles that spring immediately to mind are:

leader, follower, non-conformist, clown, scapegoat, mother, gossip, bully, bore, baby, know-it-all, moralizer, critic, controller, supporter and stirrer.

Do any of these strike a chord for you? Do any others come to mind?

For a more formal classification of the roles people take, consider the often quoted role groupings devised by Benne and Sheats (1948). As you will see, they identify three types of roles and then offer detailed examples of the range of activities each role group encompasses.

Group task roles. The purpose of these roles being to facilitate group effort.

1. the initiator/contributor suggests new ideas
2. the information-seeker asks questions
3. the opinion-seeker asks for clarification of values
4. the information-giver offers facts

THEORY INTO PRACTICE

Exercise to consider your own role-taking

A. Working either by yourself or with a partner, think of
   three different groups to which you belong (for instance a
   family, work and social group). Reflect on the following
   questions:

   1. Are there any roles you habitually take on board (for
      example always being the leader, or the baby or the
      frivolous one in the group)?
   2. Are the roles related more to your own individual
      needs or to the demands of the situation?
   3. What factors influence your choice of such roles? To
      what extent is your role-taking influenced by your own
      inclination, rather than the behaviour of other group
      members?
   4. Which roles do you like and why? Which roles do you
      dislike and why?
   5. What makes it difficult to change and move out of the
      disliked roles?

B. Consider three groups in which you have been a leader.

   1. What roles did you play in that capacity (for instance
      energizer, information giver, coordinator, encourager)?
   2. Are the roles related more to your own individual
      personality or the demands of the situation?
   3. Is there any particular aspect of the leader role you find
      difficult?
   4. Would you say that you have the ability to take on a
      wide range of roles as a leader, that is to say, be a
      different type of leader according to the demands of the
      situation?
   5. How might you enrich and extend your role repertoire?

5. the opinion-giver states his or her beliefs
6. the elaborator spells out and expands ideas
7. the coordinator clarifies relationships and pulls threads
   together

8. the orienter considers the group's position in relation to its goals
9. the evaluator-critic compares the accomplishments of the group to some standard
10. the energizer arouses the group into action
11. the procedural technician carries out routine tasks for the group
12. the recorder writes down suggestions, records decisions and acts as the 'group memory'

Group building and maintenance roles. The function of these roles being to build group centred activities and feelings

1. the encourager praises and understands others' points of view
2. the harmonizer mediates differences between members, relieving tensions
3. the compromiser meets others half-way to maintain the group harmony
4. the gate-keeper and expediter facilitates the flow of communication and encourages others to participate
5. the standard setter or ego-ideal expresses the standards for the group to achieve
6. the group observer and commentator notes, interprets and presents information about the group process
7. the follower goes along with the group ideas and actions

Individual roles. These roles reflect attempts by members to satisfy their own individual needs which are irrelevant to the group task

1. the aggressor deflates and attacks others, expresses disapproval
2. the blocker tends to resist and be negative
3. the recognition-seeker calls attention to him or herself by boasting or acting in unusual ways
4. the self-confessor uses the group as an audience to expand on personal feelings and philosophies
5. the playboy can be cynical, nonchalant and distracting

The function of group roles

Every group member can be observed to play at least one role in any group. Often members take on a variety of roles according to the needs of the group and the contributions they choose to make. In a painting group for example, one dynamic member, Anne, is keen for the group to paint a vase of flowers and she sets the vase on a central table. She is acting as a leader. If another member, John, walks in at that moment and says in a laughing tone, 'Oh no! Not Anne's flowers again!', he is acting the roles of clown, challenger, and potential leader all at once. If eventually the group decides to paint the flowers in the garden then a further challenge arises. Someone else may well organize (lead) the equipment needed and Anne and John could find themselves carrying chairs, as directed. This group has now had at least three leaders who have adopted and changed various roles before brush has touched paint. Group roles may thus be fixed or fluid according to the purpose of the group and the events of the moment.

Roles are typically functional in that they serve either individual or group interests in some way. A work **task group** needs workers, energizers, and people who will give information and initiate decision-making. In more **social groups**, we need harmonizers, encouragers and clowns. Moreover, people adjust their role according to the roles others adopt. In a group of people who are naturally followers for instance, a leader is likely to emerge if needed by the group to achieve their task.

THEORY INTO PRACTICE

Case example – the role of the clown

Background description. The clown is a social creature who jokes around, is always ready with a quip or amusing piece of behaviour. In a group of friends this is accepted as fun and natural. In therapy situations, this behaviour may well be more significant. Often the clown takes on the function of 'a harmonizer', relieving tensions (for example by sharing laughter and so displacing discomfort). Sometimes, the role may take on a more defensive function by helping the group

---

to evade 'heavier', more painful problems. This is usually achieved by turning a potential conflict into a joke, thereby keeping the exchange superficial.

The dynamics underlying this role are intriguing. Early on in a group, the clown may joke to relieve tensions (for self and others). By becoming the focus of attention, the clown absolves the other group members of responsibility for taking the social initiative. The members are then grateful and reward the clown with positive attention, reinforcing the behaviour. The clown is then likely to become stuck with that role, as the group expects the jokes to continue. Later on, however, members may prefer another behaviour and get irritated by the constant clowning.

The pertinent question to pose about the clown role is whether the clown behaviour is a chosen response to group expectations by someone who has a rich role repertoire and could behave differently, or is it the only behaviour he or she has mastered as a defence in social situations. In the latter case, will the clown be able to relinquish the role when required? If not, he or she stands in danger of being excluded in some way.

Case example. Neil was the only male member in a work group putting together a magazine. The women in the group tended to pay him extra attention and seemed to expect him to take the lead. Neil felt uncomfortable with this expectation and lacked the confidence to lead. He found he was most able at a social level as he made the group laugh. He quickly assumed the clown role. After a time the other members wished to move onto the magazine work and became irritated when Neil persisted in clowning around. The therapist stepped in and assigned Neil to be in charge of one part of the production. This allowed Neil to save face in terms of group expectations, whilst gaining self-confidence in his leadership ability.

Problems that can arise with group roles

Problems and conflicts concerning the roles people take can arise within a group and it may prove critical to identify what is happening and why. Commonly, 'role-lock' can occur when an individual is stuck in a fixed role and stereotyped behaviour.

THEORY INTO PRACTICE

Case example – the role of scapegoat

Background description. The scapegoat role and situation is a poignant and powerful one. It is painful for the individual concerned and can signal wider group conflict. The group leader needs to be aware of the dynamics underlying this problem in order to intervene appropriately.

The scapegoat is the person who is singled out and blamed. He or she is often 'different', new or disliked in some way, and thus receives the projections of the group. Often, when a group is beset by failure, a member is singled out as the 'cause' of what let the group down. By identifying the source of failure, the group reaffirms its own worth. In psychodynamic terms, the group copes with unpleasant feelings by ascribing them to an individual who is then scorned for possessing them and rejected. Thus, we commonly find a complex interplay of individual and group dynamics is involved in creating a scapegoat situation.

Case example 1. A number of conflicts and hostilities exist in a particular staff group, although the group invests a lot in, and prides itself on being cohesive. With heightened tensions some members are beginning to argue, and some are feeling apathetic about work. One staff member who is looking for another job becomes the focus of group aggression as he is seen as lacking commitment and motivation. The feelings projected onto this member unite the staff, allow a legitimate focus of anger, and displace any guilt members have about their own apathy.

Case example 2. A group of residents are engaged in a highly competitive volley ball game. As one team begins to lose one member is singled out as the 'problem'. The team starts putting more pressure on her and she gets more anxious, fumbles the ball and feels a failure. Having this scapegoat allows the failed team to feel that they could have been a success. It is interesting to speculate how much of this role the scapegoated member subconsciously assumed in the first place as part of either being supportive of her team or in an effort to receive some negative attention.

The role is either adopted by the individual or ascribed to him or her by the group. This is a problem, as it prevents change and means that responsibility can be avoided. The scapegoat examples well illustrate this process.

'**Role-status**' is another problem which can occur, where some members occupy higher status roles and others are

---

THEORY INTO PRACTICE

How to help people take on new group roles

Occupational therapists are centrally concerned about people's roles in daily life. Often group therapy is aimed at encouraging new or more adaptive role behaviour. Consider the suggested techniques offered below which aim to help individuals extend their range of roles.

1. As a group leader, do not take on all responsibility and roles, for example, leading, supporting, clearing up, challenging, initiating. Ask for volunteers and, if necessary, allow the group to flounder in order to give other members the opportunity to step in.
2. Encourage the group to consider and discuss the roles they are playing in the group. Encourage the participants to decide if any other behaviours and roles are needed by the group. For instance, a supportive, nurturing group might realize that it would be a constructive development for the group if occasionally, more challenging and critical roles were adopted.
3. 'Role-playing' is a formal way of experimenting with new roles on a trial and error basis. A typical assertion role play, for example, could be for members to practise taking faulty goods back to a shop. Help members to feel safe enough to take the risk to try some role playing and then ensure they are given constructive feedback afterwards.
4. Suggest that an overly vocal group member act as an 'observer' to a group in order to gain a different perspective or model a certain behaviour.
5. Recognize and praise positive attempts to try out new roles, such as praising a quieter member who experiments as a challenger.

forced into subservient positions. Such hierarchical social structures, which stratify members, can result in the creation of subgroups which reduces overall group cohesion. One example of this occurred in a group of students where they were required to carry out a problem solving exercise then feed back their information to the rest of the class. Two older, experienced members took on a leadership role and delegated the more boring but central tasks to the others. When it came to the feedback session, they spoke on behalf of the group in a way that unfairly made it seem that they had done all the work.

Finally, 'role conflict' commonly occurs when individuals are forced to occupy roles which are disagreeable to them (for instance being a 'secret-holder'). If a member carries too many roles at once, the role demands may conflict and result in stress. For example, a potential role conflict is generated in psychotherapy groups when leaders are required to analyse the dynamics of a group whilst also seeking to maintain their role as feeling, participating group members. These leaders could well find it difficult at times to push away their own feelings in order to concentrate on the group.

INTRA-GROUP RELATIONSHIPS

Complex relationships always exist in groups as each member relates to every other member differently. Furthermore, these relationships can shift with time as the group goals and members' roles change. This section will explore three analytical tools which are often used to unravel these complex relationships: sociometric structure, the process of subgrouping and the dynamics of triads.

Sociometric structure

Moreno (1953) has made a special contribution to understanding the structure of a group and the inter-relatedness of members. He developed an analytical tool called the 'sociometric test' or 'sociogram'. This test simply involves asking group members to choose or reject other members according to a criterion, for instance, 'most liked'. The resulting pattern of choice gives us an insight into the underlying social structure of the group.

Moreno viewed this structure in terms of interrelationships, namely: numbers of isolated members (who neither choose or are chosen); unchosen members; mutual attractions (pairs); chains (linked choices, not necessarily mutual); triangles (mutual); and stars (chosen by many but chooses no one in return).

Consider the three hypothetical groups below which illustrate the use of the sociometric test. See if you can draw your own conclusions about the relationship dynamics of each of these, then look at my comments.

A. Members are asked to rate two people most liked in the group and this is the result (see Figure 2.1).

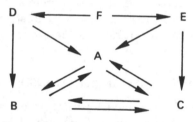

Figure 2.1 Attraction sociogram.

In the above sociogram, A is the most central, popular member, having been chosen by four people. B and C are the second most popular members. We might hypothesize that A, B and C form a cohesive sub-group or clique. D and E are the more peripheral members as no one in the main clique chooses either of them. They go along with A's popularity and select someone else in the clique as second best. Perhaps they aspire to join the sub-group and may even try to conform to its norms and values. F is the least popular member, unchosen by anyone. Interestingly, F chooses the most marginal people. This could indicate F is least identified with group attitudes and indicates either an isolated person or a non-conformist.

B. A more complicated sociogram emerges if we involve greater numbers of people. In this example, members are asked to identify the two people they would most like to collaborate with on a work task (see Figure 2.2).

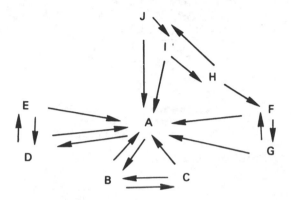

Figure 2.2 Collaboration sociogram.

In this collaboration sociogram, A is clearly a central member as eight people wish to work with him or her. H, I and J are more peripheral and largely remain unchosen by others. The most striking pattern, however, is the strong pairings which seem to form the core of three sub-groups.

Now imagine how these group dynamics would change if we knew the particular roles played by each member. Member A might be the group leader, which makes sense given the central nature of his or her involvement. An alternative scenario, which dramatically changes the picture, is that I is the group leader. This could be a potentially difficult situation if I is alienated from the rest of the group and resents A's centrality. Viewed positively, the group may operate effectively if I remains distant.

The group is likely to operate well if B/C, D/E and F/G have to work closely with each other, on the other hand, if J/B and I/A are to collaborate, the alliances may well be unsatisfactory.

C. Members in this smaller group are instructed to rate the degree of popularity of other members (see Figure 2.3).

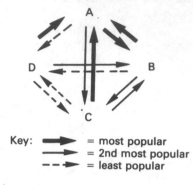

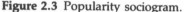

Figure 2.3 Popularity sociogram.

In the popularity sociogram above, A and B are perceived as the most popular members and D the least. It is interesting to speculate if this configuration would be similar to the individuals' perceived popularity of themselves. If A felt the least popular member, for example, the discrepancy could say something about his or her self-esteem.

These three sociometric examples demonstrate both the value and limitation of this method of understanding relationships in groups. Sociograms can give a good indication of alliances, sub-groups and the emotional position of members within a group. On the negative side, interpretations about members' attitudes and the quality of relationships are necessarily rather speculative.

This method of unravelling group dynamics is practically applied in four different ways. First, it is used as a research method to investigate group dynamics. Second, it may be employed to establish cohesive work groups where, for example, you put together the people who have chosen each other. Third, sociograms can be a powerful tool for giving insight and feedback in the therapeutic situation. For instance, ask members to compare their different perceptions of the group relationships. Finally, as a management tool it can aid in the process of establishing lines of supervision and co-leader partnerships.

Subgroups

An informal structure of relationships quickly develops in groups where members are attracted or antagonistic to each other. When members have a commonality of ideas and attitudes, they are brought closer together and may well form the sort of subgroup shown in the collaboration sociogram (Figure 2.2).

Subgrouping can be an **advantageous** process. First, having diverse sections of group life enriches the group experience and tempers any excessive demand for group conformity. We see this clearly as therapists working in a multidisciplinary team. Isn't it best to have some debate in the team rather than everyone conform to the viewpoint of one person, for example, the consultant? Second, subgroups can be a source of strength and support. This is especially important for quieter members, or those daunted by the larger group. The sub-group can act as a stepping stone for new members who need a slower introduction to a group, but note this only really works if the informal subgroup broadly reinforces the formal group aims and values. Third, sub-groups enable groups to organize them-selves to tackle a wider range of tasks and to work more efficiently. A carpentry group may send one sub-group to find wood and another to prepare the workshop, whilst a third sets about designing the item. This may be three times as fast as all working together on every task. Similarly, if several indi-viduals in a group need one-to-one activity it may be possible simultaneously to pair members and achieve different goals in each sub-group pairing.

Subgrouping also has its **disadvantages** and can be a destruc-tive process. Members' identification with their sub-group may be so intense that it detracts from their allegiance to the group as a whole. Further, sub-groups may function as competing cliques which can impair group cooperation. Consider the situation where a decision making committee is made up of two powerful and antagonistic cliques. Views are likely to be polarized in support of one camp or the other and consensus decisions will be hard to reach. This type of group dynamics interferes with the effective functioning of any committee.

THEORY INTO PRACTICE

Destructive subgrouping

In a therapeutic community establishment every resident belonged to one of several work groups which carried out the daily living tasks of the community. A destructive process emerged when one work group began to feel a stronger allegiance to their subgroup over and above the community needs. They began to work against the community philosophy. At first it showed in small things such as charging 'outside' residents higher prices for their produce. Later, a more serious problem for the community emerged when the sub-group began to question the authority of the wider community and favoured their own committee rulings. The situation degenerated until the main leader of the sub-group left the community. Subsequently, it became clear that this leader, a staff member, had felt in competition with other staff members and had used the subgroup as a way of exercising more power and status.

Triads

The triad is a special type of sub-group and has been studied in some detail. The interaction and relationship between three people is a relatively simple pattern to conceptualize, yet it captures rich relationship dynamics.

In the late 1950s, Haley (1976) introduced triads into the study of families. He made the useful distinction between 'alliances' (two people in agreement or who share a common interest) and 'coalitions' (two people united through criticism or concern for a third). Consider the configurations below and see how these concepts are applied. Whilst the examples relate to family dynamics, they can be applied equally effectively to general group situations.

A.      All these people are in agreement. This is a stable, cohesive group arrangement.

B.   One pair agrees and each of them disagrees with a third. The best example of this configuration is to place Z as a child in argument with two united parents (XY).

C.   One pair is in conflict whilst they each agree with the third person. X's agreement with Z is threatened by the Y-Z relationship. A marital therapist is typically in this situation between two warring partners.

D.   There is conflict and disagreement all around in this configuration, that is typical of a disengaged, conflict-ridden family.

Key: 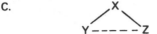 ————— = agreement
        −−−−−−− = disagreement

Figure 2.4 Triad configurations.

THEORY INTO PRACTICE

A family therapy view of secret coalitions

Two examples drawn from the field of family therapy based on systems theory illustrate how the analysis of triads is used in practice.

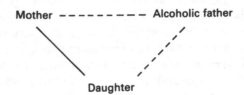

Figure 2.5 Family therapy triad.

Mother and daughter have entered into a secret coalition in conflict with the father, who has an alcohol problem. Mother and daughter's complaints about excessive drinking may increase the father's sense of exclusion and may perpetuate the situation. The family therapist might well aim to re-assert the generational boundary and strengthen the partnership between mother and father if possible.

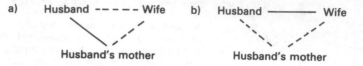

Figure 2.6 Shifting triads.

The dynamics between family members shifts dramatically between these two alternative scenarios. In example a, husband and wife are in conflict. Husband and his mother have a relationship which excludes the wife. We could speculate that the mother-in-law is the cause of the marital tension. In b, husband and wife are united by their disagreement with mother — a configuration which may well help to sustain the marital relationship.

INTERACTION

Complex verbal and non-verbal communications occur throughout every group as members interact. These interactions are complicated, as the communication can take place at a conscious and unconscious level simultaneously. Also, the communication never stops — even if people ignore each other they will have communicated their lack of interest!

We can try to make sense of these interactions in different ways. This section explores interaction in groups by focusing on: a) task versus social communications, b) the verbal content alone, and c) the overall pattern of communication. Any interaction which occurs in a group can be analysed using these three methods.

Task versus sociable groups

Every group displays task-related interactions and social interactions. Groups which aim to achieve something (such as a work activity) will involve greater levels of task related inter-action. Members will talk about the task, make decisions and problem-solve together. Groups where members chat and share their feelings display more social and emotional inter-actions. While the balance between the task versus social aspects shifts according to groups aims, both elements can usually be observed in all groups. A person may be part of a work group but also find the friendly relationships with other members satisfying. Alternatively, a group of friends can meet socially, yet may also seek to pursue some specific goal.

Argyle (1967, p 126) developed the following matrix to describe interactions in groups involving task and sociable activities (see Table 2.1).

Argyle's work is interesting because it gives theoretical rationale for, and useful insight into, the way we use task groups to achieve therapy goals. Argyle expresses the intel-lectual and social requirements of both the task and sociable activities demanded by a task group. It is precisely these requirements which we seek to identify and exploit when we design a therapeutic programme for a patient or client. Thus a casual visitor to a gardening group might only identify the therapist as involved in the verbal task of explaining the process of how to take a cutting to the members. In reality the therapist is also facilitating and monitoring a range of behaviours. He or she will watch for signals from group members that they understand (non-verbal/task). The group will chat, share their thoughts and experiences (verbal/social). The therapist will also encourage members to participate by smiles and nods (non-verbal/social).

Table 2.1 Task versus sociable activities and motivations

	Task	*Sociable*
Verbal	Information and discussion related to the task	Gossip and chat, jokes and games, discussion of personal problems
Non-verbal	Task performance, help, N V comments on performance, N V signals conveying information	Communicating interpersonal attitudes, emotions, self-presentation

Verbal interaction

Bales (1970) and his colleagues at Harvard University Social Relations Laboratory, developed a set of categories to classify communication behaviour in groups. The system is known as 'Interaction Process Analysis'.

Bales categorizes observable interaction into its task and social–emotional aspects. **Task orientated** contributions are sub-divided into two main groups concerned with giving, or asking for, information, opinions and suggestions. The **social–emotional** behaviours are sub-divided into positive and negative contributions according to whether they advance or inhibit emotional support and cohesion. There are 12 categories in all (see Figure 2.7).

A further dimension of Bales' model is the concept of equilibrium in group interaction. Behaviours can be viewed as balancing pairs (see key a – f in the table). Positive interactions complement and may counteract those which cause disharmony, fragmentation and insecurity. Negative social emotional reactions (group D) need to be balanced by positive ones (group A), and contributions requested (group C) need to be answered (group B). Heap discusses this mutual dependence in terms of systems theory, and regards the continuity of a group as 'dependent upon a reciprocity of interaction contributions – any actions or comments calling forth complementary reactions and re-adjustments from others.' (Heap, 1976, p 115)

Bales' interaction process is often used as an observational tool in research to analyse people's communication in groups. A common finding is that individual participation is a function of: group size, personality, status in the group and knowledge and physical location within the group. People also differ in their type of communication. Thus, high participators tend to give information and opinions, and speak to the group as a whole. Low participators, on the other hand, tend to contribute more by asking questions or expressing agreement and direct these more to individuals than to the group.

Another finding revealed by Bales and others is that those who contribute more also receive more messages from others. This pattern cascades down to the least productive members, who tend not to receive any communications at all. This pattern of unbalanced interaction can become fixed in a group

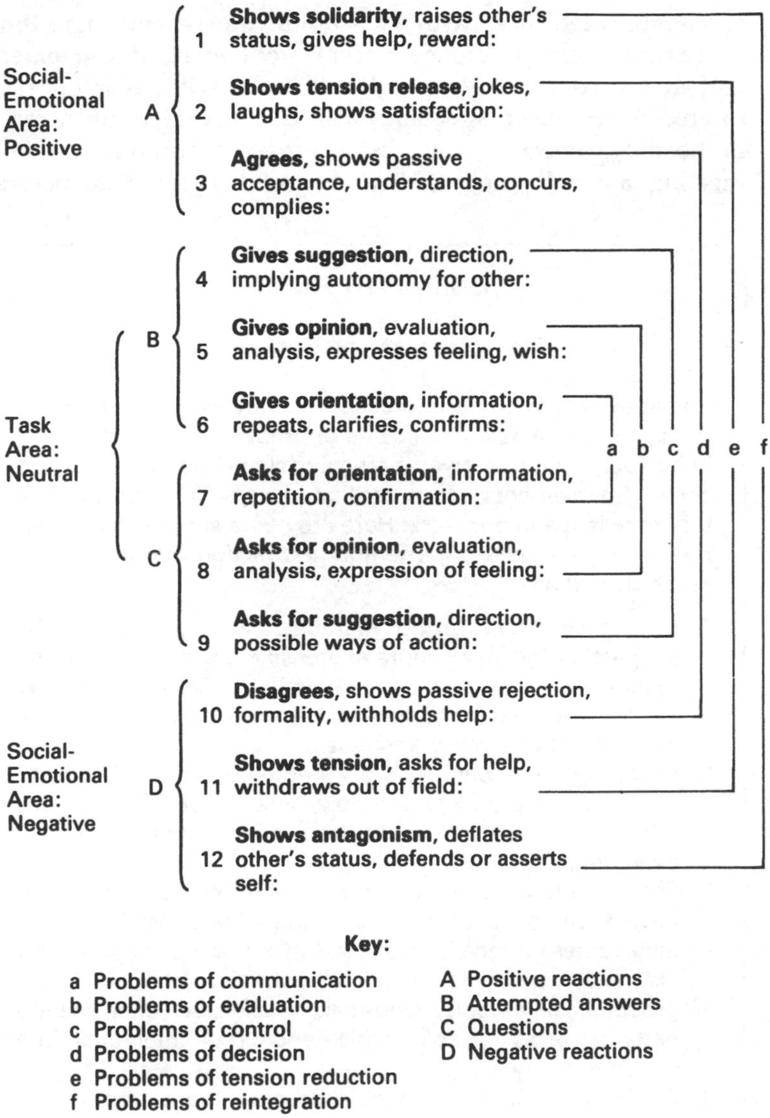

Figure 2.7 Bale's Interaction Process Analysis.

where one or two individuals receive disproportionately high degrees of attention, with the majority of communications being addressed to them.

Other studies, such as Heinicke and Bales (1953), show that

as members feel safer with each other, they spend more time expressing feelings, are better able to tolerate disagreement and are less conciliatory towards each other without an increase in anxiety. Heinicke and Bales also demonstrated an increase in hostility, rejection and disagreement around the second meeting, a development that can be seen as part of the natural

---

THEORY INTO PRACTICE

Applying research on interaction to practice

The above research on interaction is relevant to occupational therapy practice as it enables us to predict certain patterns of behaviour in groups given particular circumstances, and also shows the elements which facilitate interaction. We can use this knowledge in our work. Here are some suggestions about how to encourage group member interaction based on these research findings:

1. Encourage silent group members to communicate by suggesting they try simply expressing agreement with the opinions of others, or ask questions. Explain that they are not required to come out with anything profound or original – take away that stress.
2. Encourage members who are beginning to participate to speak to the group as a whole, instead of to individuals (often the leader). This furthers group involvement for everyone.
3. Forestall the development of rigid patterns early on, where only a minority of members participate. Wider group involvement might be achieved in a number of ways, for example: use smaller group/pair activities within the larger group; have an early ice-breaking exercise; alter seating patterns; or assign roles which encourage interaction in a structured way.
4. Check that across the whole session the expression of negative feelings and disagreement is balanced sufficiently by agreement and positive feelings.
5. Where relevant, assign group roles to members or give them a sense of having a function in the group. Electing a leader can ease conflict more quickly, particularly in task and decision-making situations.

evolution of a group. It is interesting to note that these groups did not have an assigned leader and conflict continued longer in the groups which did not agree a leader.

Patterns of communication

Another way of understanding the interaction which occurs in groups is to consider the wider, more structural, methods of communication. The quality of communication which occurs in any group, or indeed any organization, is fundamentally dependent on members having the opportunity to communicate.

Below are three patterns which conceptualize different communication networks. Note how the available channels of communication affect our capacity to function, how we get frustrated if we feel unable to participate, and what happens when the lines of communication break down.

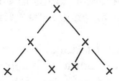

Figure 2.8 The hierarchy.

In this model the communication channel operates through a hierarchy. Decisions are made at the top and passed down, ideally after having received any relevant information from the people below. This pattern commonly occurs in Occupational Therapy departments where we have a Head, Seniors, Basic Grade and Support Staff.

Figure 2.9 The circle.

The members of this group or organization operate on an equal access and sharing basis. This model is commonly adopted in Community Mental Health Teams where members of the multidisciplinary team communicate freely with each other and leadership circulates.

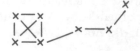

Figure 2.10 The clique.

The clique represents more complex communication networks where a central group of people are in close contact and others are isolated with limited access to information. This can be applied to many units. It is clearly seen on wards where the doctors and nurses are in close communication but other disciplines, relatives and even the patient may be unsure of decisions made.

The above are only some kinds of communication networks occupational therapists encounter. Can you think of some others?

In our real work situations, a combination of the above patterns often operates along with some others as illustrated in Figure 2.11. In the first example, (a), the hierarchy and circle together represent an effective treatment team pattern where the consultant has a specific coordinating role whilst other members can communicate freely. In example (b) a clique and a line are combined to represent a common pattern where rehabilitation departments (possibly a clique as a result of geographical proximity) have to communicate with the doctor through the ward nurses.

There is no one ideal pattern of communication network. The choice of communication channels depends on the structure and needs of the organization, group or group activity involved. Some units may function best operating where the channels of communication are in a hierarchy and the leader takes responsibility for seeing decisions through. In other groups a more democratic configuration is needed. The crucial issues are the effectiveness of the network relationships and how they cope when the lines of communication break down. In situation (a) (Figure 2.11), for example, what happens to the teamwork if the consultant is a poor communicator, or if the weekly ward round (the one opportunity for the team to meet as a whole) is missed? In example (b), what happens if a

a. Hierarchy and circle

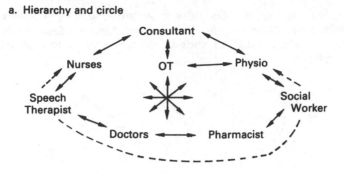

b. Clique and line

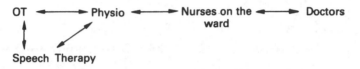

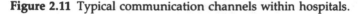

Figure 2.11 Typical communication channels within hospitals.

message between the therapists and doctors is lost between nurses on different shifts?

THEORY INTO PRACTICE

Patterns of communication experiment for the classroom

This experiment is based on one conducted by Bavelas (1950). Students, the subjects of this experiment, should sit in chairs laid out in the relevant patterns. They each assume a role with its accompanying restricted communication channel as illustrated in Figure 2.12 below. Each member is given (secretly) a card with a different symbol on it. Out of six possible symbols, one is missing. Care must be taken to ensure the students do not communicate (verbally or non-verbally) outside their permitted channels. The experimenter times how long it takes for one group member to discover which symbol is missing. Each member then describes his or her feelings about the task. Compare the results of each configuration in terms of its efficiency and the level of satis-

faction experienced. Consider how the results would have
shifted had other communication lines been in place. Apply
the modelled restricted lines of communication to real life
situations.

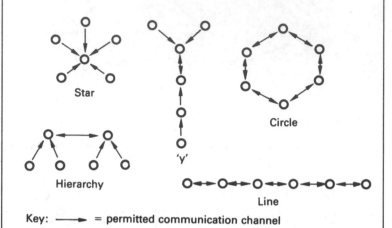

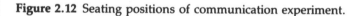

Key: ———▶ = permitted communication channel

Figure 2.12 Seating positions of communication experiment.

The result you can usually expect with this experiment
(providing nobody cheats!) is that the circle configuration
offers the greatest satisfaction levels whilst being relatively
inefficient (slow). The star is usually fast, but members often
feel dissatisfied and uninvolved. The Y, line and hierarchy
produce a range of results depending on what happens to the
communication and who takes responsibility. Predictably the
core people are more active, so feel satisfied (or pressured!)
whilst the peripheral members feel more apathetic.

NON-VERBAL BEHAVIOUR

Verbal behaviour is only part of how people communicate with
each other. A whole series of non-verbal behaviours, such as
body movements, expand or contradict our verbal communications. Non-verbal behaviours are important because they
can be a powerful means of communication, one that is often

unconscious rather than under individual control. It is vital that group therapists are aware of these communications – both our own signals and those from others. We should know our own non-verbal behaviour in order to be able to use it well. We must be able to interpret sympathetically signals to us from group members who may well have social problems precisely because they lack awareness of their own non-verbal communications. Further, when running a group we need to watch for and understand non-verbal communication occurring between members. There is a huge volume of this type of communication flowing at all times in all groups and it is impossible for anyone to absorb it all. However, the better we understand the elements of the behaviour, the better chance we have to interpret and intervene appropriately. Table 2.2 below, classifies and summarizes types of non-verbal behaviour under four headings – physical, body motion, spatial and vocal.

At a **physical level** we communicate attitudes and feelings through our appearance, posture and touch; for instance, a person sitting in a slumped, withdrawn posture is communicating a level of dejection or depression. The way we **move our bodies** like nodding, facial expression, gesture, gaze and eye contact gives off a range of signals; head nodding, for example, is a key way that we encourage others and affirm what they are saying – watch to see how often it happens in a group! Our **spatial behaviour** is less obvious to most people but we all have our own sense of personal space and always position ourselves deliberately in relation to others; for example, if someone comes up very close to another it can be an intimate, or a threatening, move. Finally, the **vocal aspect** of our speech, namely, tone, timing and stress, are a crucial supplement to our verbal messages; thus someone might say he or she feels

Table 2.2 Range of non-verbal behaviours

Physical	Body motion	Spatial	Vocal
appearance	nodding	orientation	speech tone
touch	facial expressions	territoriality	timing
posture	gesture	proximity	stress
	gaze	positioning	
	eye contact		

confident about carrying out an activity, but say it in such a hesitant manner that it is clear the reverse is true.

Non-verbal behaviours have three main roles in communication: 1) **To support verbal messages** – for example, non-verbal aspects can change the meaning of words; also they are used to control and synchronize speech. 2) **To communicate emotions and attitudes** – people give and receive feedback and share things which cannot be expressed through words. 3) **To substitute for speech** – when speech is impossible, for example when people are handicapped, then sign language, mime and facial expression take over.

Whilst all aspects of non-verbal behaviour are pertinent to group situations, I have selected three key examples – eye contact, touch and positioning – to illustrate the rich significance of non-verbal behaviour.

Eye contact

Eye contact has four main functions. First, we tend to establish eye contact as a signal that we wish to initiate interaction, though we look away when we begin to speak. Second, we look at a speaker about 60% of the time while listening, whereas while we talk we look at the listener approximately 30% of the time. Third, the more we look whilst talking, the more likely we are to be believed and accorded influence. Finally, prolonged gaze implies greater interest in the person speaking than in the content of what is being said. Findings such as these emphasize the importance of eye contact in groups (Argyle, 1967).

Both the quality and the quantity of eye contact have significance. If eyes are focused on the speaker in a group this may indicate listening and interest, whilst boredom or lack of interest is signalled if people look away. If a listener's eye contact is prolonged, it may convey a critical evaluation of the speaker's contribution, or it may suggest some sort of challenge. If the speaker attempts to gain eye contact, this may be a way of inviting response or support, alternatively it may be an attempt to provoke. Avoiding eye contact may be evasive or indicate a wish to be excluded or conceal emotions. It may also be an expression of feeling bored, threatened or guilty.

As group leaders, we need to be aware of our own eye

contact to ensure we include all members in face-to-face contact. This is a skill that requires practice, but it is crucial if we want to communicate interest, recognition and support for all the members of the group. Moreover, we can use our eye contact effectively to encourage one person to speak and to discourage others.

THEORY INTO PRACTICE

The use of eye contact to influence behaviour of others in a group

To illustrate how eye contact may be employed to influence another's behaviour, consider the situation where a group member over-monopolizes the conversation. The other members are likely to avoid any eye contact and will minimize other encouraging non-verbal actions, in order to control the one-way flow. Hopefully, the over-dominant speaker will pick up these cues. If not, the leader or another member might employ eye contact in order to indicate the wish to interrupt. If that does not work, then someone just has to interrupt, verbally!

Touch

Touch occurs relatively infrequently in groups, at least in Western cultures – so why discuss it in preference to other behaviours? The reason is that when it does take place, touch with all its ritual and taboo can be extremely powerful. It can be lovely, warm, comforting and therapeutic. Conversely, it can be dangerous to use, especially when it is misinterpreted, or perceived as offensive or invasive. We are all likely to touch others in a therapeutic situation but before doing so we should reflect carefully on its possible impacts.

The touch that occurs in our social world can be classified along a continuum of: functional (clinical/purposeful); social (polite/pleasant); friendly (warm/caring); and intimate (close/ sexual). In our different groups, the functional and friendly type of touch will occur most frequently. Functional touch tends to take place during activity groups, and usually involves the therapist touching the patient or client to direct or demonstrate an action. Also, it naturally occurs between members, say in a sports group. Friendly touching, where people comfort, protect, care for or appeal to each other, takes place in the context of relationship-building therapeutic groups.

How and when touching occurs in a group is, not surprisingly, influenced by the social and cultural norms of society at large. In much of Western society, for instance, touch between women and men, or women and women, would appear to be more acceptable than that between men and men. This has been communicated strongly to me in drama therapy groups where men often seem ill at ease touching each other in sensitivity exercises. These same men had less trouble when lively or aggressively friendly touch was called for. It is interesting to note that groups can evolve norms for touching which are at variance with wider cultural norms. Individuals, for example, who would not normally choose to hug each other, can suddenly find themselves hugging group members unselfconsciously and with enthusiasm in a group game!

Research shows that touch can influence individuals. In a review of the literature, Hargie *et al.* (1981) conclude that touching can help individuals to talk more about themselves and their problems and that individuals are more likely to comply with requests and favours when touched. The uses of touch to facilitate behaviour or disclosure is a powerful tool in therapy – and this is an area where we must particularly guard against being too manipulative or abusing our power.

Touch is used in two deliberate ways in occupational therapy group situations. There is the use of touch in normal interaction, and then we may deliberately encourage touch through exercises. Therapists use touch to encourage and assist patients or clients. When this has a functional, clinical purpose, such as lifting, the touch is usually accepted easily. When we use touch with individuals in a group to show support, or to console, we need to be more careful. Thus, for example, when someone starts to cry we might proffer a gentle, spontaneous hug to comfort, and when the boundaries within professional relationships create barriers and prevent the use of such touch it may be acceptable to encourage other group members to take on this role. However, it is important to note that some people dislike being touched and feel invaded rather than consoled and this must be respected. We also need to recognize that using touch as a 'pat-on-the-back' can be experienced as patronizing rather than reassuring.

Touch exercises and group games are often used to promote group bonding and trust. We may also encourage the use of touch in massage or other exercises for relaxation. These more structured ways of using touch need to be handled sensitively and developed gradually. It is counter productive to force intimacy. Thus hand massage is considerably less threatening (hence more relaxing) than body massage.

THEORY INTO PRACTICE

Grading touch in drama therapy

Consider how the level of touch demanded in these group games is graded by time and intimacy.

Game	Touch
'Wink swop'	Accidental
'Hug tag'	Exuberant but selective
'Group sculptures'	Cooperative and functional
'Rag doll/tin soldier'	In pairs and in play
Sensitivity exercises	More intimate and prolonged

Discussion questions

1. In what ways does culture influence our use of touch in groups?
2. To what extent does a group leader's use of touch shape group norms?
3. Should a group member who dislikes touch be allowed to 'sit out' of group exercises involving touch?
4. In your view, when would the use of touch be undesirable in a group?

Positioning

Where and how people choose to position themselves (to sit or stand) in a group can give information about their relation-

THEORY INTO PRACTICE

Some problem seating positions – reasons, effects, solutions

What would you do if you were the leader in these two situations where the seating positions may pose a problem? My suggested responses are offered at the end of the box.

1. During a group activity, two members, E and F, have elected to isolate themselves at another table (see Figure 2.13). The main group have not particularly offered them sufficient space. Equally, you suspect that E and F may be asserting their stronger allegiance to each other over the group. Should you insist that E and F join the bigger group, given that the aim of the session is to promote group interaction?

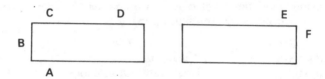

Figure 2.13 Isolated positions.

2. A new group member asks you if he can work alone at a table as he feels nervous when close to others in a group. The aim for him in attending the activity session is to develop his work skills. Would you agree to this request?

Suggested responses:
1. How about putting the two tables together? If this is not possible, invite (more welcoming than insist!) them to join. If they are still reluctant you might let it pass for that session but take the opportunity before the next to discuss with them the treatment aims and the importance of working together.
2. Yes, if it does not interfere with the group activity. This is the first session and the member may need a gentle introduction to the group. Subsequent sessions would be a different matter.

ships, motivation and feelings at that time. Moreover, the position chosen can, in turn, affect the group interaction. Imagine the situation where a patient attends a group discussion, but elects to sit outside of the discussion circle, slightly away from the other members. The patient may be saying he or she does not want to be part of the group and is withdrawing, possibly as a protest or because he or she feels bored or threatened. By adopting what is in effect an observer role, the patient may well affect the rest of the group, for example, by being a distraction as they wonder what is the matter. Alternatively, the members themselves may have subtly excluded the patient by not making extra room.

In a detailed analysis of the effects of seating positions, Heap (1977) has reviewed the research literature and describes five observed 'regularities'. (Note that he refers particularly to discussion type groups where members sit in a circle). First, members who are more highly motivated or who want more attention seem to place themselves near the leader. Second, those next to the leader may get 'forgotten', so the leader needs to make extra effort to ensure they are in the field of vision. Third, the seat farthest away from the leader is often initially attractive to unmotivated or insecure members, though being directly opposite the leader (common term is 'hot seat') is most exposed. Fourth, if members change seats it is significant, for instance, motivated members may be shifting away from the leader to achieve better eye contact. Finally, the 'hot seat' is often taken over by more motivated, aggressive or dominant members.

Research shows that where people sit in a circle individuals interact most with people opposite them and interactions reduce progressively as people get closer. Thus in Figure 2.13 below showing a circle of ten people the speaker interacts least with people in positions 1 and most with those in position 5. The arc displayed is called the field of greatest interaction and occurs in the position equivalent to 3.6 placings in a group of ten people (Steinzor, 1950). In practical terms this means that we can facilitate involvement and participation of quiet people in groups by sitting them together opposite expressive ones.

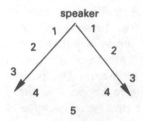

Figure 2.13 Field of greatest interaction.

DECISION MAKING IN GROUPS

As therapists we are regularly involved with making decisions in groups. Within our therapy groups we encourage patients and clients to take part in deciding which activity they would like to do or how to execute it. In staff meetings we take decisions concerning unit policy or decide whether to pass or fail students, and of greatest importance, in multi-disciplinary team meetings, we decide patients' or clients' futures. When a group decision has to be made some complex dynamics emerge.

The decision-making process

The process of making decisions in groups characteristically involves four phases. The group may glide smoothly through each phase, or it may move back and forth within them. The first phase is **planning** and this is where the problem is identified. Members ask questions such as, 'What do we want to achieve?', 'How should we approach the task?'. In the second phase of **exploration**, the parameters of the problem and solution are discussed. Brainstorming ideas is a technique that is particularly useful here as the group is opened up to creative possibilities. In the third phase of **judgement**, the pros and cons of each solution are evaluated and different group members will usually give their opinions. Finally the **decision making** occurs and a solution is agreed. Unanimous decisions are hard to achieve in less cohesive groups or in groups where members do not share many values. In this case a consensus or majority decision may be reached.

Group decision making requires **participation** and **consensus**. All group members need to feel free to state their opinions, and discussion should enable people to explore the options. After open discussion the decision made should reflect members' opinions rather than a leader imposing his or her view. Without this process, the decision made is not a 'group decision'.

THEORY INTO PRACTICE

Some examples of group decision making

Here are three examples of decision making. In your view do they reflect effective and desirable group decision making processes? Why? Discuss these different scenarios with some colleagues. Do you all agree?

1. In a ward round all the multi-disciplinary team members, bar the consultant, argue strongly against a particular treatment. The consultant, who has overall medical responsibility, chooses to give the treatment anyway.
2. A group of patients cannot agree on where to go for a community outing. The argument is mainly between two people who wish to go to two different places. After a lengthy discussion the occupational therapist suggests that the group goes to one place this time, and the other next time.
3. In a staff meeting, members are trying to formulate a new policy. They are uncertain of their ground but discuss a range of options. The team leader has additional, relevant information but remains silent until the discussion has run its course. When the team leader gives her opinion, the rest of the staff agree.

Often a group is not able to come to a decision or solve a problem. Consider the following four examples of how group dynamics can interfere with the decision-making process. Firstly, the members may be worried about the consequences of the decision, such as fearing the absent leader may not sanction it. Similarly, if members are comfortable with things as they are, groups may never find a solution as they may fear responsibility, change or failure. For example, one staff group could not come up with topics to be included in the weekly peer group teaching session because members were reluctant to set themselves up to teach.

A second example of group dynamics interfering in the decision-making process occurs as a result of interpersonal difficulties between members. Conflicts between members or sub-groups may ensure views are polarized and consensus never reached. One group member may be particularly negative and veto all suggestions.

A third obstacle to the decision-making process may arise when members have conflicting loyalties between this and other groups. Occupational therapists are frequently in this position, as they straddle two sometimes opposing groups. An illustration of this is the occupational therapist who works in a multi-disciplinary team. As a team member he or she may wish to discharge a patient because of pressure on beds, whereas as a therapist he or she may wish the patient to remain for further treatment.

Finally, tensions can build in a decision-making group when some members desire unanimous decisions and do not accept the principle of majority rule or consensus. Given this, it is a good idea to estabilsh the type of decision making required before embarking on the process.

Research on decision making

Lewin (1984) pioneered much of the early work on group decision making. In one study he investigated how housewives could be persuaded to change their food habits, for instance, buying cheaper cuts of meat. He studied the effectiveness of presenting one group with information through a lecture and another via group discussion. He found that only 3% of the lecture group changed their habits as compared with 32% of those who participated in group decision making. This kind of study demonstrates the power of group processes in shaping behaviour.

Research on decision making has revealed some specific processes at work here, the most common of which are 'group polarization', 'risky shift' and 'group think'.

Group polarization. Do you think decisions made by groups and committees are likely to be more conservative or more radical than an individual's decision? Research backs up both results. Moscovici and Zavalloni (1969) suggest that often members become more extreme in their decisions in a group, but only in the direction of the original inclination – hence the term 'group polarization'. The old adage that decision making by committee results in conservative decisions applies here, but only if the committee members start off in a conservative frame of mind, otherwise the opposite result would occur. An example of this is when a supervisor feels unsure about whether or not to fail a student on fieldwork experience and discusses this with colleagues. If the colleagues believe the task of failing a student should not be shirked, the supervisor is likely to be moved in this direction.

Clark and Keeble (1987) review the literature and explain this phenomenon in terms of: a) diffusion of responsibility – that is to say, it is easier to take a more extreme position when no one individual assumes responsibility for the consequences; b) information sharing and persuasive arguments – through discussion, members have additional information available with which to make a more definite decision; c) 'social comparison theory' (Festinger, 1954) – individuals want to present themselves in the best possible light and often the adoption of risk is assumed to be socially desirable. When caution is seen to be more socially desirable, the decision made will be more conservative.

Risky-shift. One interesting example of group polarization is the risky-shift phenomenon, first noted by Stoner (1961). His basic experiment (see Theory into Practice box below) demonstrated that group discussion generally resulted in higher risk choices compared to the choices the individual members had made previously.

Group think. Group think is a phenomenon described by Janis (1972) where members in highly cohesive decision-making groups strive for unanimity. Critical evaluation of ideas takes second place to consensus and facts or views which oppose the preferred policy are 'swept under the carpet'. Members wish to maintain 'group morale at all costs and to do nothing to spoil

THEORY INTO PRACTICE

The risky-shift experiment

Try your own group decision-making discussion using the following choice dilemma taken from Stoner's experiment. First, decide as individuals what level of risk you feel is acceptable, then have a group discussion and come to a consensus decision. What happens?

Mr B, a 45-year-old accountant, has recently been informed by his doctor that he has developed a severe heart ailment. The disease would be sufficiently serious to force Mr B to change many of his strongest life-habits, reducing his work load, drastically changing his diet and giving up favourite leisure-time pursuits. The doctor suggests that a delicate medical operation could be attempted, which if successful, would completely relieve the heart condition, but its success could not be assured, and in fact the operation might prove fatal.

Imagine that you are advising Mr B. Listed below are several probabilities or odds that the operation will prove successful. Please tick the **lowest** probability that you would consider acceptable for you to advise* that the operation should be performed.

- Place a tick here if you think Mr B should not have the operation, no matter what the probabilities.
- The chances are 9 in 10 that the operation will be a success.
- The chances are 7 in 10 that the operation will be a success.
- The chances are 5 in 10 that the operation will be a success.
- The chances are 3 in 10 that the operation will be a success.
- The chances are 1 in 10 that the operation will be a success.

*Note that this is a fictional exercise taken from Stoner's experiment. As professionals, we would never directly advise on such an issue. Instead we would help Mr B come to his own decision.

the comfortable "us feeling"' (Clark and Keeble, 1987, p 46). In all, the internal pressure to conform, along with limited discussion, means that the decisions made are questionable. Group think is likely to occur when: a) a decision-making team is close and has to continue working together; b) the group is isolated from others; c) the group is under some external threat; d) the members are influenced by a strong leader who is able to promote his or her views.

Discussion questions

1. Make a list of decision-making groups you participate in at work. Do the groups have any characteristics in common? Are they effective in their decision-making?
2. Is majority rule a fair way of making decisions?
3. Have you experienced 'group think' in any group? How could it have been avoided?
4. In a decision-making group what would influence you to change your position?

B. Case examples and analysis

In this section the group dynamics of two different groups are described then analysed. The first is a pottery group and its focus is on the task at hand. The second group, called the 'next step group', is more psychodynamically orientated for contrast. Neither group is particularly unusual or outstanding. I have selected these 'routine' groups to emphasize that all groups are eventful.

As you read the description of each group, try to analyse what is happening and why. Break down events described into the elements of activity discussed earlier in the chapter and see how this helps you explain the observed behaviour. Note too how it gives more objectivity to your interpretation. Then look at my brief analysis to see if we have picked up similar points. You may well find that we have drawn different understandings from the data, so do not be concerned if you have noted something different. There are no absolutely right answers to group interpretations, though there are better and worse ones.

EXAMPLE 1 – A POTTERY GROUP

Background

The pottery group meets every Tuesday afternoon in the Occupational Therapy Department of an acute admission psychiatric unit. The aim of the group is to encourage basic and unpressured social interaction of people who are isolated, socially anxious or demonstrate poor social skills. The group was set up as a semi-open one, where members are encouraged to come regularly in order to feel more comfortable in the group and to build relationships.

Members

The group has seven members, including the occupational therapist, but attendance of any one member on any particular day is unpredictable. The group has three long-standing members, two of whom attend regularly, while others come and go depending on their mental state and needs on the day. Being an acute admission unit, it is not uncommon to have a new member join the group while another is discharged. The members who attended on this particular occasion were:

John, a regular attender, is a shy, middle-aged man who lacks confidence in his abilities and is anxious in the company of others.

Susan, a long-standing but inconsistent attender, is a young woman who has had a severe schizophrenic breakdown and finds it difficult to relate to other patients. She remains somewhat childlike and often demands much staff attention.

Dave, a fairly new member, is a depressed, withdrawn, apathetic young man who had been admitted for acute anxiety during the exam time at his art college.

Mike, a regular attender, is a man in his late twenties suffering from a recurrent manic–depressive illness. In addition, he has cognitive/perceptual problems resulting from a head injury 2 years previously. His concentration remains poor and he tends to be unaware of others' needs.

Marjory, a new member, is a middle-aged woman who was admitted to hospital with a problem of benzodiazepine abuse.

Example 1 – a pottery group 55

She is now on a withdrawal programme which leaves her tense and irritable with others.

Sheila is the occupational therapist and group leader.

Summary account of the session

John arrived first and sat quietly to wait for the others. Sheila used this opportunity to ask him if he was finding the contact with others in the group any easier. He replied that he was, but still felt unable to start up any conversation with anyone and felt easiest working by himself.

Susan then rushed in, unaware of interrupting, and asked Sheila if she had to do the pottery today as she was feeling unwell. The ensuing discussion revealed that Susan had been upset by the ward round held that morning when she was told she was not yet ready for discharge. Having 'off-loaded' her feelings and gained some encouragement, she was content to sit down.

At this point a nurse brought Dave into the room – he did not attend on his own initiative. Sheila greeted him, and as the nurse left, asked Dave if he wanted to be in the group today or whether he preferred to stay on the ward. Dave agreed to stay and joined the other two sitting around the large central table – the signal for Sheila to start the group officially.

Sheila began by showing the members the now glazed pieces of pottery fruit they had made the previous weeks which had been combined together in a large fruit bowl to become a group sculpture. Susan and John were particularly pleased with their efforts. Sheila then suggested they might have a go at the pottery wheel this week – something none of them had tried before. All three members were a little unsure, but agreed. As there was only one wheel, Sheila asked with an encouraging smile who was going to go first. John agreed to do so; as usual he was hesitant, but wishing to cooperate with whatever is asked of him.

While Sheila demonstrated the basic technique, holding her hands around John's against the turning clay, she explained the process to all three members. The other two watched with increasing interest. John soon relaxed and was clearly enjoying himself. He eventually worked independently and created a creditable first-attempt bowl. By this time, Susan was keen to be involved and pushed her way between Sheila and John, asking to be next. Sheila commented on her intrusive behaviour and suggested Susan ask the others if they minded her being next. Sheila sorted out a new piece of clay and centred it for Susan (the more technically difficult job). She then directed John to teach Susan as he had been taught. Whilst they worked together, Sheila talked quietly with Dave, asking about his experiences in watching the wheel in use at his art college.

At this point, Mike raced in, talking cheerfully, if somewhat incoherently, due to his slurred and pressured speech. He exclaimed over the fruit and then again over the activity at the pottery wheel, which made everyone smile. Sheila greeted him and said he would have to wait for a while before it was his turn and would he like to do something else in the meantime? Mike agreed, as without a concrete activity to keep himself focused, he became restless. She sat at the table with him and together they worked on some more fruit pieces (his request).

Sheila re-centred the clay for Dave to have his turn. He quickly picked up the technique from John and worked independently. John and Susan joined Mike at the table, sharing their pleasure about what working with clay on the wheel was like.

Another therapist appeared at the door and introduced Marjory to Sheila. Marjory was clearly tense and said somewhat resentfully that she had not really wanted to come. She had never done pottery before and probably would not be able to do it now as her hands were very shaky. Sheila acknowledged Marjory's uncertainties and suggested she just try out this one session and then decide whether or not to come back. She also suggested that if Marjory was reluctant to work with the clay, she was welcome simply to watch what the others were doing. A calmer, less reluctant Marjory agreed to stay.

Sheila introduced her to the group members and suggested she watch Dave for a while if that was agreeable to him. After a few minutes she was encouraged to have a turn and experiment with the clay. Initially, she proved adept at shaping the clay, but then she suddenly became frustrated and smashed the newly created bowl shape which had begun to get a bit wobbly. She shouted out that she could not do anything – it was hopeless and her hands were too shaky. Dave immediately

Example 1 – a pottery group   57

intervened and encouraged her to try again. Together, they re-created a bowl from the remains of the damaged one.

The rest of the group progressed in a similar pattern with pairs working together either at the table or on the wheel. John continued to guide Susan, while Dave encouraged Marjory. Sheila was left to 'contain' Mike who periodically amused the group members with his clumsy antics and jokes. Over the space of an hour each member created several clay items.

Towards the end of the group Sheila drew all the members around the table to discuss what they thought of the pottery session. Everyone seemed to have had fun and were pleased with what they had produced. Unanimously they asked to repeat the wheel activity the following week. Sheila agreed, asking if everyone would be there. Susan piped up that she would come if John helped her again. John was pleased. Marjory thanked Dave for supporting her and said she was surprised at herself but found she would also like to come again.

Analysis of the group processes

Roles

Sheila was very much the group 'leader'. She was directive in that she selected the activity and made suggestions for how members might become involved. She actively encouraged each member to be involved, responding to their individual needs. She took a more nurturing role with Susan, Marjory and Mike, whilst responding in a more adult-to-adult way with John and Dave.

John and Dave interestingly adopted a sort of 'co-therapist' role, helping and teaching Susan and Marjory, respectively. Perhaps this occurred in response to Sheila's higher expectations of them?

Susan appears to have adopted a 'child-like' role where she receives extra tolerance and attention from the 'adults'.

Mike acted as 'group clown', which is a role that offers him a positive function in the group, thus compensating to some extent for his limited task and relationship skills.

Marjory went through several roles and phases from being an 'outside aggressor' to 'the emotional one' where she was fairly 'self-orientated' to becoming more 'group-orientated' at the end.

Relationships

The sociometric structure of the group relationships might be represented something like that shown in Figure 2.14 below.

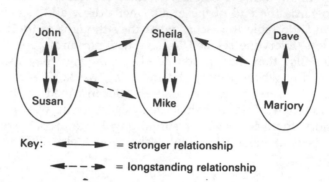

Key: ◄────► = stronger relationship

◄─ ─ ─► = longstanding relationship

Figure 2.14 Sociogram of relationships within the pottery group.

The group evolved into three working pairs which gave strength and support to each individual. Relationships developed within each sub-group more than within the group as a whole. The relationship between John, Susan and Mike might be predicted, as these three are long standing members.

Interaction

This group involved greater levels of task-related, as opposed to, social and emotional interaction. It is interesting to note how the nature of the task – being satisfying for some and frustrating to others – led on to social and emotional interactions.

The interaction between the group members could be displayed using an interaction sociogram such as in Figure 2.15. It is interesting to note that this sociogram reveals a star type pattern.

Bales' Interaction Process Analysis can be used to highlight the type of interaction most frequently observed. Table 2.3 summarizes some key points.

Example 1 – a pottery group 59

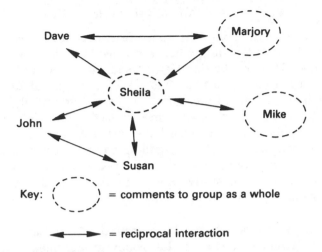

Key: comments to group as a whole = comments to group as a whole

= reciprocal interaction

Figure 2.15 An interaction sociogram of the pottery group.

Table 2.3 Summary of interactions using Bales' Process Interaction Method

	John	Susan	Dave	Mike	Marjory	Sheila
shows solidarity	✓	✓	✓		✓	✓
shows tension release				✓		
agrees	✓					
gives suggestions	✓		✓			✓
gives orientation						✓
asks for opinion						✓
asks for suggestion		✓			✓	✓
shows tension		✓			✓	

Three features of the group are strikingly revealed by this summary table. One is that many of the interactions are in the positive socio-emotional or in the neutral task area. This can be seen as evidence for the overall positive 'feel' to the group. A second feature is that there is a similarity of interactions between John and Dave, and these complement Susan and Marjory's similar interactions. Thirdly, Sheila inevitably interacts at several different levels, which represents her high level of input to the group.

Non-verbal aspects

The main non-verbal behaviour described in the case study is that of hands touching when the wheel technique was demonstrated. This may be significant, as touch can be either a source of tension or comfort. In this instance it seemed to be more positive, as none of the members were close initially, yet they all tolerated the more intimate contact within the context of the activity. This may well have increased the bond between members, aiding trust and enabling group cohesion to develop.

It is worth noting that while no specific reference was made to it in the case study, Sheila probably used a great deal of listening and encouraging facial expressions and body positions.

Finally, the seating position around a large table may well have facilitated some of the wider group interaction. Conversely, the close proximity of the pairings undoubtedly encouraged their interaction.

Discussion questions

1. In this type of group, should the aims be acknowledged openly? Were they?
2. The group met around the table at the beginning and end of the group. What purpose was served?
3. What roles did Sheila, the therapist, adopt and why? Could she have selected a better approach?
4. Sheila worked on a one-to-one level with Mike and had one-to-one contact with the others at several points in the group. In this instance was she justified or might it have been counter-productive?
5. An end product appeared to be an important element of Sheila's choice of activity. Do you agree that this was necessary for this group?
6. Do you think that the kind of analysis that we have just engaged in aids understanding or provides any ideas about how to improve our groupwork practice?

Example 2 – a support group 61

Decision making

The main decision-making function lay squarely on Sheila's shoulders. She made the rules, selected the activity and to a large degree controlled the members' behaviour. The group members did have the opportunity to make some choices and could come to their own decisions about what to make. Crucially, some group decision making emerged at the end when members made commitments to attend together the following week.

EXAMPLE 2 – A SUPPORT GROUP

Background

The following example takes a short excerpt from discussion which occurred in a women's support group called 'the Next Step Group'. The women have met weekly for an hour for the last 6 weeks. The group is planned to carry on as a closed group for two more sessions for which the women have contracted to attend. The aim of the group overall is to consider the 'next step' towards building up new ways of coping.

The members

The group consists of six women, including the therapist. All the members have contributed to the group on different occasions; they have shared their difficulties and offered support to the others. Each member has different problems, but they have all lost an important life role recently, leaving them stressed or distressed.

Dorothy, the main protagonist in this scenario, has recently 'lost' her daughter and her mother role (Dorothy's daughter and son-in-law emigrated to Australia). Dorothy has an alcohol problem and her husband is a compulsive gambler.

Excerpt of one session

Dorothy started off the group by sharing some of the difficulties she had faced over the week. Tearfully she related a number of annoying incidents concerning her husband, who had lost quite a lot of money gambling. Finally she says with determination, 'I'm going to leave him. We've been married 30 years. I've wasted the best years of my life on him, I'm going to leave him.'

Rachel, the therapist, interrupted this monologue: 'You've now told the group a number of times that you will leave your husband. I'm not so sure I accept that you want to do this.'

'Are you saying you don't believe me?', returned Dorothy, prickling defensively.

Rachel nodded her response.

Brenda retaliated on Dorothy's behalf, 'That's a foul thing to say! I know what it's like to live with a difficult husband. I wanted to leave mine for years. Dorothy needs a medal for what she has put up with.'

Anita supported Dorothy too. 'Why did you say that, Rachel? That's quite hurtful.'

'At that moment, I just felt strongly, Dorothy, that you don't really want to leave your husband – in a funny kind of way you need him, warts and all', responded Rachel gently.

Dorothy quietened, 'I don't know what you mean . . . the way he treats me . . . He never gives me enough housekeeping, spends all his earnings betting on the horses . . .'

Anita intervened, stemming Dorothy's fresh flow. 'I think I understand what Rachel is saying. You need him to blame and have someone to let your anger out on. Where would you be without him? What would you do? It's not that you're lying. The feeling of needing to stay with him is inside you, without you knowing it in your head.'

'Yes' agreed Rachel, 'somehow you gain something from your marriage'.

Dorothy was now puzzled. 'I don't see that I gain anything – apart from headaches. What am I gaining?'

'What does everyone think?' Rachel responded. 'Can we help Dorothy here?'

After a pause, a calmer Brenda suggested 'Security maybe? Better the devil you know and all that?' She looked at Rachel for confirmation.

Rachel did not reply immediately. She then mused, 'I wonder if it's also something about you being able to carry on drinking as long as your husband makes no effort to change? This way you let yourself off the hook.'

Example 2 – a support group 63

Analysis of the group processes

It is, of course, impossible to offer a full analysis of the group process on the basis of using just a few minutes of conversation. To understand a group fully, you need to be able to observe it and experience it at several levels. The following notes on my analysis simply indicate the likely direction of the group and are offered as an illustration.

Roles

Rachel's therapist roles are supporter, confronter and group observer.

Dorothy takes a self-confessor role. She is in danger of adopting a victim stance, but later becomes a positive listener.

Brenda is initially an aggressor to Rachel and an encourager of Dorothy. Later she becomes an initiator–contributor.

Anita acts as a harmonizer mediating differences, and a gatekeeper facilitating the flow of communication. In these ways she can be seen as the co-therapist for this part of the group.

Relationships

A dynamic set of alliances and coalitions are apparent in this short excerpt. First, Brenda supports Dorothy in a coalition against the 'punitive' therapist. Anita in turn allies herself with the therapist but supports Dorothy by showing she understands. Thus Anita defuses a potential conflict. (Figure 2.16 illustrates these two situations using a triad analysis.) Rachel then unites the group by asking everyone for help in support of Dorothy. This eases the tension between them and draws Brenda back constructively.

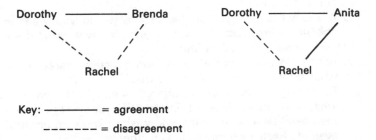

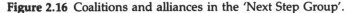

Figure 2.16 Coalitions and alliances in the 'Next Step Group'.

Table 2.4 Interactions within the 'Next Step Group'

	Dorothy	Brenda	Anita	Rachel
shows solidarity		✓	✓	✓
agrees		✓		✓
gives opinion				✓
gives suggestion		✓	✓	
gives orientation	✓			
asks for opinion			✓	
asks for suggestion	✓			
shows antagonism	✓	✓		

Interaction

If we analyse each intervention made according to Bales' inter-action process analysis, the findings might look like Table 2.4.

Non-verbal aspects

The only data we have on non-verbal aspects of this group relates to the indications of attitude and tone of voice indicated in dialogue text as 'gently' or 'puzzled'. We could surmise that the group is seated in a circle and that a wide range of emotions and attitudes will have been displayed by members.

Discussion questions

1. Would it have been as helpful if Rachel had adopted a less confronting role?
2. If you were a leader of this group, would you want to encourage members to openly disagree with you? If so, how would you achieve this?
3. Rachel describes herself as a non-directive therapist. To what extent do you think this is true?
4. Reflecting on the analysis offered earlier in the chapter, what additional kinds of information about the group members' behaviour would you wish to know, in order to evaluate Rachel's interventions further?

Example 2 – a support group 65

Decision making

None apparent.

This chapter has explored group dynamics by examining the group processes concerned with roles, intra-group relationships, interaction, non-verbal aspects and decision making. The first section outlined the theory, the second section applied the theory to practice using two case study examples and analysing their group dynamics.

Describing a group through its processes can be a helpful and relatively objective way to understand group dynamics. However, the essence of the group may not be fully captured. Sometimes, we need to look to other factors such as the current theme and atmosphere of the group and appreciate the changing nature of a group's involvement. These elements we explore further in the following chapter.

3

Group dynamics: the evolution of a group

Groups that come together regularly over a period of time change and develop. They evolve through certain stages and experience identifiable feelings, preoccupations and behaviours as they develop. These stages are not necessarily sequential, nor will all stages be experienced by every group. A group may miss a stage or return to an earlier one, and stages can overlap where behaviours normally associated with different stages occur within the same group. Despite this, every group faces certain developmental issues as part of its ongoing dynamics.

Section A of this chapter explores the different **stages** through which a group can be expected to evolve. Then two group processes particularly associated with a group's evolution – **norms** and **cohesion** – are considered. Section B illustrates how the theory can be used in practice by giving a summary account and analysis of one particular social skills group which took place over the course of 10 weeks.

A. Stages, norms, cohesion

STAGES OF A GROUP

Different theorists conceptualize the stages of a group's evolution differently. This section describes the views of Tuckman, Shultz and Mosey, and sets them in the context of support and activity groups as shown in Table 3.1. Four 'Theory into Practice' boxes then show how a therapist can facilitate a group's development through its various stages.

Table 3.1 Stages of a group – different theorist's views

Support group	Activity group
Tuckman = forming storming norming performing	Mosey = orientation dissatisfaction resolution production
Schultz = inclusion control affection	terminal

Support group stages

Tuckman (1981) encapsulates the developmental stages of psychotherapy groups in the terms: forming, storming, norming and performing. In the **forming** stage, members ask questions. What are the purposes and rules of the group? What am I supposed to do? Do I want to be here? Will I fit in? This is a period of orientation, anxiety, testing and dependence which we have all experienced when we have joined any new group.

The **storming** stage is a time of intra-group conflict. The group members feel a lack of unity and a resistance to the group task. They may express hostility to the leader or therapist for not solving the problems and the leader's competency may be directly questioned. Issues of power and control versus withdrawal or dependence are raised.

In the **norming** stage, strong norms and a group culture emerge. There is a cohesion between members as they disclose more and work together to resolve conflicts. It is a time of closeness and the group tends to be self-preoccupied.

In the **performing** stage, the group works more actively on achieving its goals and energy shifts away from forming the group towards the job at hand. Members trust and support each other and they are able to express constructively both positive and negative feelings.

Schultz (1958) takes a different approach to stages of group development and discerns recurring emotional themes of inclusion, control and affection. Group interaction is predominantly related to one of these dimensions. The **inclusion** stage is characterized by developing relationships. Members want to belong, yet are uncertain and test the boundaries. The **control** stage involves problems of competition and cliques. Individuals establish roles in terms of power and status. The **affection** stage is one of pulling together and trusting in each other. The group appreciates its uniqueness and identity. Schultz views these stages in cyclical terms, with themes repeating and reversing as the group moves towards ending.

Activity group stages

With reference to activity groups, Mosey (1986) describes five discreet phases: orientation, dissatisfaction, resolution, production and terminal. In the first **orientation** phase, members are eager to be a part of the group. They have positive expectations and some anxieties about the unknown. This is a time to get to know group members and test the boundaries of the group. Members tend to be dependent on the leader, other members or the activity. Mosey suggests this phase is shorter if the group has a specific structured task to achieve.

The **dissatisfaction** phase is characterized by intra-group conflict and high emotional expression. Group members are confronted by the reality of unmet hopes and begin to feel uncomfortable with their dependency on the leader. Sub-groups emerge, negative feelings are expressed and work on the activity at hand decreases. The resolution of this phase depends on how easy it is to work through frustrated feelings and get on with organizing the activity (which in turn may need to be redefined to be more achievable).

The **resolution** phase begins with the decrease of dissatisfaction. Members now feel more positive about themselves and take pleasure in doing the activity. Norms and cohesiveness develop, roles are defined more clearly and work on the task increases. The **production** phase continues this positive process. Members roles become more flexible and functional. The group knows what it is doing, can mobilize its resources and resolve internal conflicts.

The **terminal** phase begins to be faced when the activity or group is ending. The group becomes concerned about its end and the movement of members into other groups. There is a sense of impending loss and anticipatory mourning. Members may also assess the success and failure of their group experience. If the group can end with a sense of accomplishment, positive feelings will be stronger than the negative ones. Work on the activity will be at its height at the beginning of this period and then will gradually diminish.

Facilitating group development

However the group stages are conceptualized, any group will have some manner of beginning and end, and in the middle, the group is likely to experience both difficult and productive moments. If occupational therapists are to be effective as leaders, it is crucial we are aware of the developmental process and needs of our group. Understanding the stages helps us to identify relevant needs and behaviours of individuals and ensures we have appropriate expectations of our group. Moreover, we can facilitate the progress and appropriate resolution of each stage.

In the **early stages** of a group the leader will want to set the scene and clarify aims and methods, create a group bond, and encourage members to participate and interact. When the group goes through a time of **confusion and conflict**, the therapist needs to keep restating aims and methods, helping the group to develop realistic expectations and a group identity. Members may need to be encouraged to use the group more, to take some risks and share material. Whilst this is a difficult time for the facilitator, he or she needs to 'hang on' and encourage honest communication whilst containing the negative feelings and keeping the group safe. As the group becomes more **cohesive and productive** in performance, the facilitator needs to encourage the group's responsibility, involvement and risk taking. The leader should offer less direction and more feedback. In the **ending stage**, the leader must be clear about when the group is to end. The group may need help to acknowledge feelings and any unfinished business. Rituals to facilitate the ending, such as a last exercise together, are important. A follow-up or reunion session at a later date may help the group to look forward.

THEORY INTO PRACTICE

Facilitating group development
Early stage*

Aims	**Example methods**
1. to clarify structure, aims and methods of group	a) have pre-group interviews b) leader might outline some typical events c) all members, including leader, should share their expectations
2. to encourage interaction	a) name games such as throwing different shaped imaginary balls to another whilst calling out member's name b) exercises which encourage members to be active and involved, for example, movement games or each member is required to say one thing c) encourage pairs and trios to work together, then build up wider interactions, for instance, pairs talk to each other then each introduces partner to the group
3. to create a group bond or identity	a) regularly use words like 'we', 'us' or 'our group' b) emphasize what is special or different about the group c) emphasize similarities of experience and needs of members, such as, each member saying one thing wanted and not wanted in the group at the start

*Forming (Tuckman) and Orientation (Mosey)

THEORY INTO PRACTICE

Facilitating group development
Confusion and conflict stage*

Aims	Example methods
1. To help members to express tensions	a) acknowledge the feelings b) as leader, try not to be defensive and stop the emotional expression c) ask other members how much they share a particular feeling
2. To keep group safe and contain negative feelings	a) be accepting of negative feedback b) leader may need to referee or end an unproductive argument
3. To encourage realistic expectations of group and leader	a) re-state aims and methods b) challenge how realistic members are being c) may need to re-define task so that it is more achievable
4. To attempt to maintain the group bond despite natural fragmentation	a) point out any 'group feelings' b) emphasize experiences shared by members c) confront group about pulling in opposite directions d) compare the needs of individuals to the common group need

* Storming (Tuckman) and Dissatisfaction (Mosey)

THEORY INTO PRACTICE

Facilitating group development
Cohesion and performance stage*

Aims	Example methods
1. To maintain group identity and cohesion	a) use exercises and games which depend on group cooperation and trust, such as trust exercises or a group painting

	b) encourage exploration of group processes such as norms, interaction, group themes
2. To encourage members' involvement, sharing and feedback	a) ask for the group's feedback regularly
	b) make links between member's comments and reactions
	c) encourage members to help each other within tasks and exercises
3. To encourage members to take the initiative and responsibility for their own actions	a) challenge members to speak for themselves for example, 'owning' the feedback they give out
	b) when asked advice as leader, demonstrate respect for the members and group, by turning it around to 'What does the group think?'

* Norming/Performing (Tuckman); Resolution and Production (Mosey)

THEORY INTO PRACTICE

Facilitating group development
The ending stage*

Aims	Example methods
1. To encourage expression of feelings such as sadness or achievement	a) recognize underlying feelings
	b) allow group to be angry or sad etc.
	c) ask members what each will miss
2. To encourage 'ending rituals'	a) have a 'last exercise', possibly one that is a group favourite or one that brings the group together such as a 'group yell'
	b) possibly give each group member something to take away, for instance a sheet of paper with compliments on it written by other members in a group exercise

	c) plan a finale such as going to the pub or having an ending tea
3. To encourage evaluation of the group	a) ask members to say what they have gained coming to the group
	b) encourage members to say how the group or activities could have been made more useful, that is to say, gain some feedback to improve methods for the future
	c) encourage members to reflect on how they have developed or changed
4. To acknowledge any unfinished business	a) establish future goals for individuals
	b) consider support systems for the future
	c) plan a follow-up day or session if relevant

* Terminal (Mosey)

NORMS

The function of norms

Group norms are the value system of a group. They order and organize behaviour, enable group members to feel safe and aid the achievement of goals. Given that every group is made up of individuals, each with their own personalities, skills and opinions, the emergence of norms is a crucial process. Applbaum *et al.* (1973) describe this process as follows, 'As group members interact, they tend to standardize their activities to create customary ways of behaving that the whole group can recognize as norms. A group norm is the shared acceptance of a rule prescribing how members perceive, think, feel and act.'

Different types of norms operate depending on the group. First, there may be many and varied norms governing members' general behaviour, such as appearance, participation and rituals like making tea at the start of the group. Second, norms about task or work behaviour evolve concerning the rate, method and standard of work which is accepted by the group.

One group may pride itself on working efficiently, whereas another may approach the task in a desultory fashion. Third, norms regulating interaction concern the content and style of typical conversation: how the leader is treated, how much emotions are expressed, how members react to a group silence, to name but a few issues. Fourth, norms relating to shared attitudes and beliefs may arise both as a prerequisite for the group (such as holding a particular political view) or they may evolve naturally (for instance, believing the group to be 'the best').

THEORY INTO PRACTICE

Norms in your staff group

What are the norms of your staff group? Here are eleven questions to ask in order to discover some of them.

1. Is there a dress norm, for instance smart but casual and never jeans?
2. Is there a punctuality norm? When, for example, do staff members tend to arrive in the morning?
3. What is the work-level norm? Is it to 'work hard'? 'Do the minimum'? Or is it up to individuals?
4. Do staff members socialize with each other or is the norm only to have a working relationship?
5. Is the head seen as an equal member of the team or as someone apart from it? How is this demonstrated?
6. In what ways does the staff group typically handle a member leaving?
7. In staff meetings, what norms are evident? What type of information is covered and by whom? Is discussion encouraged?
8. Does lunch time conversation tend to cover work or non-work related topics?
9. What is the norm regarding modes of address? Are some staff referred to by their titles, for instance, 'Dr'?
10. How much touch is used between staff members? Is it acceptable to hug each other in comfort or celebration?
11. How far are individual members allowed to 'deviate' from any of the above without attracting disapproval?

Some group norms can conflict with each other and this can create tension. A group may aim to be 'caring and supportive' but evolves a norm which suggests that an individual should not ask another how he or she feels. In this case the norm is at odds with the goals of the group. At a wider level, a group's norms may conflict with that of the wider community, for example, being allowed to express freely suicidal ideas in the group – something that may be less acceptable outside.

Norms evolve in every group as members decide what is acceptable and unacceptable behaviour for the group at any point in time. This decision making process may occur at a verbal level where rules are discussed. It can also occur at a non-verbal level where people model on each other and respond to cues signalling approval or disapproval. If a member does not act in accordance with the norms, he or she will be subject to sanction by other members. This can take the form of telling the person he or she is wrong or punishing the member in some way, such as ignoring or dismissing the person from the group. Members mutually socialize each other through this subtle process of norming.

Norms can help or hinder

Norms are necessary for a group to function. First, they offer safe and acceptable ways of behaving which serve to increase the predictability of the group. In order to feel safe in a group situation, we need to know what we are supposed to do and what everyone else is likely to do. Without this knowledge, we are likely to feel threatened and the group will be 'unsafe' – our experience when we join an unfamiliar group of people. Second, norms allow the group to work towards achieving group goals. Norms which emphasize group cooperation and effort are usually helpful here. At the very least, it would be inefficient to have to re-negotiate the ground rules constantly, such as who is to suggest the activity for the day. Third, norms can act as a powerful defence for the group. In a psychotherapy type group, for example, norms will evolve about safe ways to express feelings which might include focusing on stresses external to the group, thereby avoiding here-and-now issues.

Whilst conformity to shared values and common practice

carries a number of advantages for a group, it can also be detrimental to the group's functioning. A group may become too defensive and institutionalized, stuck in certain patterns of behaviour. This reduces the creativity and life of the group and narrows its viewpoint. This can be seen frequently in staff groups which have had the same personnel for several years.

THEORY INTO PRACTICE

Problem situations of unhelpful group norms

1. In a projective art group, there was an expectation that members would first paint, then discuss their paintings. In her first session, one client felt unable to describe her painting. This was a critical moment as the therapist needed to weigh up the advantages and disadvantages of allowing this deviation from the norm. On one hand, allowing the client to opt out of this exercise would demonstrate sensitivity, understanding and willingness to hand over responsibility to the members about how they wish to act. On the other hand, it risked allowing a 'non-disclosure norm' to develop. If other members copied it, the projective activity would be sabotaged effectively. On this occasion, the therapist accepted the silence but asked if she could 'speak for' the client. The next time round the therapist directed the client to say just one thing, thereby reinforcing the norm of sharing material verbally.
2. In a creative writing work group, the members were spending an increasing time chatting and drinking coffee, and less time on writing. Social rather than work behaviour was becoming the norm, contradicting treatment aims. The therapist was forced to review the goals of the group with the clients and become more directive about prompting work behaviour. This continued until the members could once again enforce work norms themselves.
3. Staff in one unit had become casual about attending the weekly meeting on time. The head of department resolved this situation by offering the staff the possibility of both starting and finishing later. Needless to say, a new punctuality norm came into being!

COHESION

The value of group cohesion

Cohesion refers to the degree of connectedness and closeness members feel towards each other and the value they place on the group. Members have a clear sense of belonging to, and belief in, the cohesive group. In a low cohesive group, members are more distant and critical.

When individuals join or leave the group it is of little importance to the members as ' the group' has less meaning. In a highly cohesive group, members interact well, are warm and loyal to each other and they trust the group. The high level of cohesion provides a sense of security, thus enabling risk-taking (such as trying out new behaviours) and self disclosure to develop.

On the negative side, a cohesive group has influence over its members which may not be helpful. The more cohesive a group, the more there are pressures to conform to group norms. This problem may be aggravated if the norms are 'deviant' (like those in gangs of soccer hooligans) or 'unhelpful' (such as those not to disclose feelings in a psychotherapy group). Too cohesive a group can result in members becoming so attached to each other that their outside interaction is limited – a problem for groups in hospital.

A number of studies support the importance of cohesiveness in group therapy. Dickoff and Lakin (1963) categorized patients' explanations of the curative factors in their group psychotherapy experience. Over 50% considered the mutual support the most helpful. Those who perceived the group as cohesive attended more sessions, experienced more social contact with others and found the group therapeutic. For those who rejected the group, the reverse findings occurred. An experiential group study by Clark and Culbert (1965) concluded that the quality of member-to-member relationship is a prime determinant of individual change. Yalom (1975) cites more evidence and extrapolates that cohesion is primarily therapeutic as it increases group attendance and participation, raises self esteem by gaining approval from valued members, allows expression of hostile feelings and increases influenceability.

THEORY INTO PRACTICE

Assessing cohesion

One way of assessing a group's cohesion is to observe individuals' behaviour in the group. In particular, look for behaviour indicating affiliation to the group such as cooperating and coordinating as opposed to withdrawing and judging. Gough (1957) suggests an exercise where an individual's behaviour can be placed along two dimensions: dominance/dependency and high affiliation/low affiliation (see Figure 3.1). Whilst an individual's behaviour rarely falls into one category, often a pattern of behaviour emerges which may be relevant.

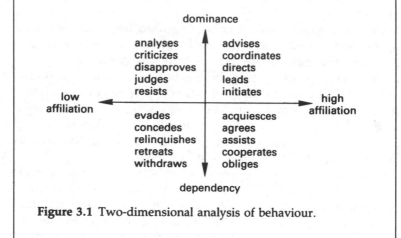

Figure 3.1 Two-dimensional analysis of behaviour.

The affiliation dimension in this context reflects the degree to which a person wishes to get on with others in the group. An individual who displays a number of the behaviours in the bottom-right quadrant, for example, would be someone who is eager to please and conforms to the norms set by more dominant members. Someone whose behaviour largely falls in the top-left quadrant would feel more distant and unconcerned about the opinion of others in the group. (Priestley and McGuire, 1983).

Developing group cohesion

Group cohesion can be developed in a number of ways. It cannot, however, be forced or artificially induced. The following strategies merely offer a possible direction which may work effectively in your group.

a) First, use of words is important. Use 'we' words rather than 'I' words, and speak to the group rather than to individuals. Note the contrast between starting a group saying, 'This is our group, we can take it in any direction we want and do any activity the group suggests.', as opposed to, 'I want you to contribute your own ideas for activities, to go in the direction you would like.'

b) Create a 'group climate' that respects members' feelings and opinions, in order to encourage the open expression of both positive and negative points. A 'storming' phase of critical comments about the group or leaders is usually a necessary preparation for a more productive 'performing' stage.

c) Make group goals explicit, which in turn emphasizes a group purpose and identity. It will also reduce the tensions which tend to arise if members do not know what they are doing.

d) Openly invite individual's participation early on, trying to prevent any members getting stuck in observer roles. Exercises which encourage everyone to be involved (such as introducing your partner to the group) are helpful here.

e) As a leader, it might be possible to model and reinforce self-disclosure and risk-taking behaviour (for instance, we might act 'silly' but not get embarrassed whilst doing a drama-therapy exercise). As these behaviours increase, so will closeness.

f) Foster member to group interaction rather than member to leader. If as leader you are asked a question, ask, 'What does the group think?' It may also be relevant, to encourage (by non-verbal gestures) members to look at the whole group when they are speaking rather than directing comments to you.

g) Try and make the group attractive and enjoyable to individuals so that they want to be there. You might, for example, have enjoyable warm-up and close-down activities to balance the more serious main section of an experiential group.

h) Use activities which foster interaction and cooperation with members. Some ideas are: group mural, trust exercises, a special outing, sharing tools/equipment, working together on a longer term project.

i) Use activities which foster a sense of commonality between members which helps people relate to each other and feel connected. Activities which involve noting similarities of attributes, interests, ideas and experiences are all useful.

j) In talking-based groups, encourage a here-and-now focus where people share their reactions about each other, with each other. This is in contrast to the type of group-distancing conversation such as monologues like 'what I did 5 years ago'.

k) Have frequent meetings. Time and predictable patterns build bonds.

l) Finally, friendly competition with other outside groups can increase the cohesion of 'in-groups' as people pull together for 'their team'. Be careful of this one though, as some people dislike competition and it can backfire.

THEORY INTO PRACTICE

Summary of how to build group cohesion

a) Use 'we' rather than 'I' words
b) Encourage open expression of ideas – positive or negative
c) Emphasize group identity with group goals
d) Invite early participation
e) Model and reinforce self disclosure and other risk-taking
f) Foster member to group interaction
g) Try to make the group seem attractive and enjoyable
h) Use activities which foster cooperation
i) Use activities which foster a sense of commonality
j) Encourage a here-and-now focus
k) Have regular and frequent meetings
l) Foster friendly competition with outside groups

Example 3 – social skills training group 81

B. Case example and analysis

In order to give a flavour of an evolving group, a social skills group involving eight consecutive sessions is described below. These eight sessions constitute a short period of time in the life of a group and as such, any change that occurs remains tenuous. As you read through the account of the group member, try to note relevant points about the stage of the group, emerging norms and group cohesion. Then compare your analysis to mine.

EXAMPLE 3 – SOCIAL SKILLS TRAINING GROUP

Background

This social skills training course consists of eight weekly sessions. The focus of the course is 'assertion'. The group takes place in a community unit and is run by two therapists (Clive and Hayley). Six clients who suffer from social anxieties and low self-esteem attend the group. The members are well motivated to work on their assertion difficulties and all have had previous experience of therapy groups. All the members have had two pre-group interviews with the leaders to assess their particular needs.

Organization of the sessions

Each group session lasts for one and a half hours and adopts the format of: warm-up game, theory discussion, role play, problem-solving discussions and end game. The topics to be covered each week are as follows:

Week 1   Introduction to group/members/shared common problems/methods
Week 2   Aggression versus passivity versus assertion
Week 3   Standing up for one's rights (legal)
Week 4   Saying 'no'
Week 5   Disagreeing with another person
Week 6   Asserting self in relationships
Week 7   Asserting self in relationships
Week 8   Evaluation/group ending exercises.

In weeks 2 and 3, all members participate in role plays to gain experience. Thereafter, one person volunteers to role play his or her problem situation. Group members then apply any learning to their own problem.

Summary of each session

Week 1. Introduction to group/members/shared common problems/methods.
Group members are a little nervous and initially reluctant to speak. Warm-up exercises help to break the ice as members discover their concerns and difficulties are similar. The leaders, Clive and Hayley, are particularly active as they give out information and demonstrate role play techniques. Group members laugh together.

Week 2. Aggression versus passivity versus assertion.
Members divide into two sub-groups and perform a role play of 'taking goods back to a shop'. Each member takes turns playing different characters and being the observer/feedback-giver. All the members participate, even though they are slightly embarrassed.

Week 3. Standing up for one's rights (legal).
A similar format of two sub-groups role playing (this time taking faulty goods back to a shop) is adopted. Two members, Janet and Keith, are particularly knowledgeable and confident as they have had experience of working in shops. They are placed in different sub-groups so that members can benefit from their experience. They both assume dominant roles. Keith is inclined to be abrasive and members in his sub-group become slightly tense and withdrawn.

Week 4. Saying 'no'.
Liz volunteers to do a role play on saying 'no' to a friend who continually makes demands to be given a lift in Liz's car. Most group members are sympathetic, except for Janet who feels Liz should 'just refuse' and Keith who is negatively critical during role play feedback. Liz gets upset and storms out of the room saying, 'I don't have to put up with this!' Hayley follows Liz

Example 3 – social skills training group   83

out to give her support. Clive encourages the remaining group members to explore what occurred.

Week 5. Disagreeing with another person.
Liz returns to the group a little sheepishly. Keith and Janet apologize for contributing to Liz's upset. Tension is eased as the members are amused by the relevance of the topic of the day. Clive suggests it might be useful to re-play the disagreements of the previous week in a more constructive way. All the members try out the different roles. Keith and Liz work well together. The other group members praise Janet's ability to disagree.

Week 6. Asserting self in relationships.
Peter volunteers to work on his problem scenario. Peter's mother forcefully indicates to him that she expects him to visit every Sunday. He has done so for the last 5 years and feels trapped but is unable to refuse. Peter becomes a little tearful and the group members are gently supportive. The role play is successfully resolved. A deep discussion ensues where some members disclose other family pressures. The group members try, unsuccessfully, to extend the time available for this session.

Week 7. Asserting self in relationships.
Anne tries to enact a role play on telling her husband she would like to do an Open University degree. Somewhat reluctantly, she discloses some deeper marital problems in response to Hayley's questioning. The members feel rather uncomfortable with this level of personal disclosure and Janet is critical of Hayley's intervention. The group members are reluctant to continue with the role plays and use the rest of the time to speak of other matters. Clive and Hayley wonder if this reaction is tied up with the group ending the following week. Janet agrees and admits she feels annoyed that the leaders are 'ending the sessions just when the group is working so well.'

Week 8. Evaluation/group ending exercises.
Clive and Hayley lead a number of ending exercises. All the group say they have gained a lot from the sessions. Janet,

Table 3.2 Evolution of a social skills group

Session theme	Stage	Norms	Cohesion
1 Uncertainty; dependence on the leaders	orientation (M) forming (T)	Commitment to attend for all sessions	limited
2 Everyone behaves' well	norming (T)	To join in role play and discussion actively	some
3 Two members become more dominant	dissatisfaction (M)	Pattern of unequal contribution developing	some
4 Conflict expressed	storming (T)		limited
5 Warm feelings	resolution/ production (M) performing (T)		strong
6 Deep disclosure	norming (T)	To disclose and give each other support	strong
7 Resistance and some withdrawl	dissatisfaction/ terminal (M) storming (T)	Group beginning to take some control against the leaders	reasonable
8 Some bereavement	terminal (M)		reasonable

key: (M) = Mosey's stages
     (T) = Tuckman's stages

Keith and Liz express their sadness at ending. Peter admits to feeling a bit panicked at the thought of suddenly losing the group's support. At the end, all the members hug each other warmly.

Example 3 – social skills training group   85

Analysis of evolution

1. Generally this was a successful group, as all members were actively involved and several problem situations were resolved. Members still felt they had a long way to go.
2. The group was enabled to work effectively, fairly quickly, because members were prepared in advance, motivated and experienced in groupwork.
3. Group dynamics of stages, norms and cohesion did not really have time to come to fruition over eight sessions and conclusions can only be tentative.
4. The stages of the group are not clear-cut or sequential, for instance norming and performing occurred together and the group returned to conflict.
5. Cohesion was aided by emerging norms of group commitment and self-disclosure.
6. Table 3.2 summarizes the group dynamics of each session in terms of a key theme, the developmental stage, emerging norms and the level of cohesion.

This chapter has explored the idea that a group evolves and relationships change over time. On-going groups appear to move in and out of stages characterized by certain behaviours and needs in the members. As a group evolves, norms develop and the group becomes more cohesive. Members feel bonded by their group identity and shared experiences. As stronger relationships develop in any group, so does its therapeutic potential. Group therapists face the challenge of creating and leading groups to facilitate the development of positive relationships. This is the subject of the following chapters on managing groups.

Part Two

Managing groups

4

Planning groups:
preparing a session

Planning group treatment – be it preparing for a single session or setting up a longer term group – is a complicated business. Many of the procedures for running a session are applicable to both types of group, though a longer term group has extra demands. In order to prepare for a session, we have to identify and take into account the needs of our patients or clients, think through our aims of treatment, and consider how to adapt our role and activities to meet these aims. Then, we have to motivate the group members to attend in order for them to benefit from the experience we have planned. When setting up a longer term group, we also have to take a number of practical decisions about the type of group we are going to run, when it will occur and where. We negotiate issues of leadership and co-leadership, and devise procedures for referral, recording and evaluation. Then, we have to prepare our future group members and engage their commitment to attend.

This chapter explains how to prepare for the one-off session. I have selected six aspects to discuss, namely, how to: establish **aims** and **goals**; choose an **activity**; **structure** the session; use the **environment**; **grade** and **adapt** the treatment; and **motivate** group members to attend. The next chapter focuses on longer term group needs.

Both this and the following chapter offer guidelines to therapists about how to plan group treatment. Most of the content relates specifically to therapy groups, but the ideas expressed can often be generalized for use within staff groups and social gatherings.

AIMS AND GOALS

Establishing effective aims and goals is the most critical aspect of planning a group treatment session. This section looks at why it is such an important process, and then explores the broad aims of different types of occupational therapy groups. Finally, I consider the process of formulating goals – both for the group as a whole and for the individuals concerned.

The value of aims and goals

There are at least five reasons why we should formulate aims and goals when planning groups.

1. **To ensure purposeful activity**. As occupational therapists, we often feel undervalued and bemoan the fact that other professions view us in terms of 'diversion' or 'simply occupying patients'. The key difference between occupational therapy and diversion is our use of purposeful activity. 'Purposeful' means that our activities are carefully selected, planned, graded and evaluated – in other words, we have clear aims of treatment. It follows that our ability to offer a therapy through activity depends on being both specific and explicit about the aims of our work. If we are not clear about the group aims and goals, can we really argue that we are not simply occupying the patients or clients?

2. **To provide policies and guidelines for structuring the session**. Knowing what we want to achieve within a group gives us clues about how to structure a session. If our aim is to encourage sharing of feelings, we will structure the session to maximize trust and interaction. If the aim is for individuals to build work skills, then we will promote a work atmosphere and provide opportunities for the skills to be practised. If our goal is to increase decision making and use of initiative in members, we will know to reduce our own level of directiveness.

3. **To provide the criteria for evaluating the group**. The process of evaluating a group at the end involves referring back to original aims and goals and seeing how well these were met. We could have goals for example, which state, 'By the end of the art session, each person will have created

at least one picture'; or 'By the end of the discussion about the trip, a decision about where to go will have been made and members will have expressed their preferences'. In both these examples, the criteria for evaluating the success of the group are earmarked. Groups which by their nature have less well defined goals may still be evaluated in terms of whether or not aims are achieved. For instance, in a group

---

THEORY INTO PRACTICE

Monitoring a patient's progress using goals

George, a patient in a rehabilitation unit, has reduced task performance and limited interaction skills. The therapist translates these problems into specific aims and goals. These are then incorporated into an assessment sheet which both George and the therapist use to monitor his progress.

Aims and goals whilst attending directive art group:
A. To attend group consistently
 – being punctual
 – staying the full hour
B. To participate in the session's art activity
 – following basic instructions
 – until task completed
C. To work alongside others
 – sharing equipment
 – responding to questions asked

Assessment form to evaluate progress
 key: 0 = No problem 1 = Some problem
 2 = Severe problem

Goal	Criteria	Week 1	Week 2	Week 3
attendance	punctuality	1	0	0
	staying full hour	2	2	1
participation	following instructions	1	1	1
	completing task	2	1	1
interaction	sharing equipment	1	0	0
	responding to questions	1	0	1

where the aim is to build trust and enable members to express their feelings, the criteria for evaluation could be the degree of self-disclosure offered by each member.

4. **To motivate and direct the patient or client**. Occupational therapy is an active treatment which requires the patient's or clients' active involvement. They need to know what they are aiming for in the group sessions in order to be motivated to strive in a particular direction. If an individual does not realize he or she is meant to talk with more people or concentrate for increasing lengths of time, how can we expect him or her to do this? Patients or clients do not want simply to be occupied, they want to know what they are doing, why they are doing it and what they are achieving. They need to know what is expected of them and what to expect of themselves.

5. **To monitor patient or client progress**. In addition to evaluating a group as a whole, we also evaluate the progress of its individual members. Once a person is working towards specific aims and goals, his or her progress can be monitored. An individual may have a goal of 'work alongside other members comfortably'. In this example, the individual and the therapist will know when it is time to move onto a more advanced goal.

Establishing group aims

In broad terms, we can distinguish between the aims of activity groups and support groups. **Activity groups** aim to develop work skills or to encourage leisure interests. The focus of these groups is the activity which will often involve a specific end product. The 'doing' element in these groups is crucial. Typical examples of activity groups are woodwork, gardening, bingo, pottery and a swimming group.

Support groups aim to encourage members to explore feelings and give each other support. The focus of these groups is on the group process. The relationships and interactions are usually considered to be more important than the activity or end product. Typical examples of support groups are discussions, social skills training, drama therapy and psychotherapy. Table 4.1 contrasts the two types of groups and offers a selection of typical aims.

Table 4.1 Activity versus support group aims

Activity groups	Support groups
to develop work skills	to explore feelings
to encourage leisure interests	to encourage members to give
to develop task performance	each other support
skills	to gain confidence
to increase knowledge of a craft	to develop trust in other group
technique	members
to learn the use of community	to share ideas
leisure facilities	

The emphasis on task skills versus social-emotional aspects can be seen in terms of a continuum (see Figure 4.1). Some groups are firmly rooted in task-related aims and others are only concerned with emotional material. Of course, many occupational therapy groups seek to combine both to varying degrees, drawing on both task and emotional elements. This can be expressed in terms of a continuum (see Figure 4.1 below).

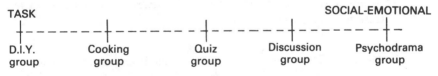

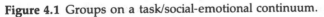

Figure 4.1 Groups on a task/social-emotional continuum.

Group aims encompass the task/social–emotional dimension. Group aims can also encompass other dimensions such as: a) 'orientation' – does the group aim to focus on an end product or the group process? b) 'development' – are the aims concerned with individual's growth or the development of the group as a whole c) 'directedness' – is the group's progress directed by the therapist or by the group members?

I find it useful to unpack and summarize group aims in terms of these three dimensions. This is best shown visually by plotting points for each dimension along a continuum.

Compare the five figures below (Figures 4.2–4.6) which contrast the aims of different groups.

1. **A work group**. The group meets regularly, working together to produce a monthly hospital magazine. The members have specific, relevant skills and established roles – a division of labour which enables them to work cooperatively. The therapist participates more than initiates. Figure 4.2 represents the aims of the group as:

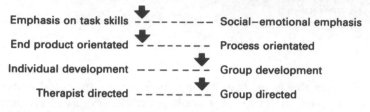

Figure 4.2 A work group.

2. **A bread baking session**. A group activity designed to be fun and encourage sharing a social interaction. Group members play together inventing different shapes for the rolls. The therapist joins in, group members contribute ideas. Bread rolls are shared and eaten at the end. Figure 4.3 describes these different dimensions:

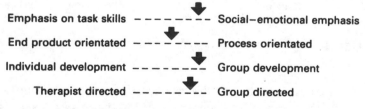

Figure 4.3 A bread baking session.

3. **A psychodrama session**. An individual protagonist enacts a painful past experience using the group for support. The therapist directs the action and encourages group cohesion and involvement. The focus remains on one group member. These different dimensions are illustrated in Figure 4.4:

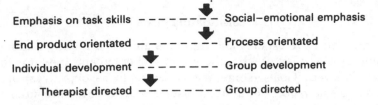

Figure 4.4 A psychodrama session.

4. **A craft session.** The therapist takes a teacher role. Having an end product is important. Individual members operate at their own level, each with their own aim of treatment. Figure 4.5 represents this as:

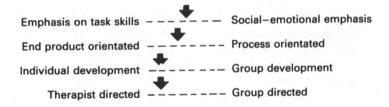

Figure 4.5 A craft session.

5. **A supportive psychotherapy group.** Members meet weekly to share feelings, make sense of experiences and to gain support. The therapist facilitates group involvement and helps the group make links between the 'here and now' and outside experiences. The group members are insightful and articulate and facilitate each other. Figure 4.6 illustrates these aims:

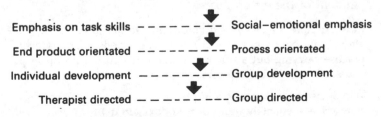

Figure 4.6 A supportive psychotherapy session.

Formulating goals

Once you have established a group's aims you require a more step-by-step plan of what the group will entail and how it is to be achieved. Goals (sometimes referred to as objectives) are precise statements of intended results, and serve as measurable targets for both patients or clients and therapists. The effective goal states what is to be achieved, how it is to be achieved and the criteria for measuring its achievement. The goals set should be realistic and agreed between therapist and group members.

Formulating the goals of a group is complicated by the fact that separate goals for both the group and the individuals may be required. **Group goals** normally state what the members will achieve by the end of the session. This is illustrated by the following two examples.

- Life skills group goals – by the end of the session, members will be able to: a) fix a new 13 amp plug onto an electrical appliance b) understand the importance of using correct fuses c) change a light bulb d) demonstrate safe handling of electrical items.
- Bread-baking session goals – members to bake and eat rolls together: a) at least three new, fun shapes to be created b) all to contribute to kneading the dough c) all members should be able to explain the recipe with confidence to others.

Goals for individuals in a group may be formulated over and above group goals as illustrated by the three case examples below. Note that in the first example, Helen's goals are specific to her and contrast with the group goals which involve encouraging members to give each other support and feedback. In the second and third examples, Fred and Mandy have goals to work on over the course of several weeks which are independent of the group goals.

Case example 1 – Helen is due to return to her job of biology teacher after a long period of hospitalization. She asked for an opportunity to practise carrying out a teaching session to a mixed group of patients and staff. Her goals for the session are:

- to devise an accurate lesson plan
- describe adequately the concept of oxygen debt
- speak clearly and confidently

– have eye contact with everyone in the room
– answer questions appropriately

Case example 2 – Fred is anxious, withdrawn and has extreme difficulty in relating to and trusting others. With help, he draws up a hierarchy of his social difficulties which in turn become his goals over several group sessions.

Goal	Criteria for achieving goal
Being in the same room as others	Be in department; feel comfortable
Having to be in close contact in the same room as others	Cope with being in enclosed room; work at same table as others
Responding to questions from the therapist	Answer questions normally
Responding to questions from other members	Answer questions normally

---

THEORY INTO PRACTICE

Example aims, group goals, individual goals for a social skills group

Aims

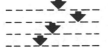

Emphasis on task skills	– – – – – – – –	Social-emotional emphasis
End product orientated	– – – – – – – –	Process orientated
Individual development	– – – – – – – –	Group development
Therapist directed	– – – – – – – –	Group directed

Group goals

1. Learn the difference between being passive/assertive/ aggressive
2. Share/disclose assertion situations experienced as difficult
3. Use appropriate assertive behaviour in at least one role play
4. Demonstrate confident body language in a role play and maintain: eye contact, relaxed, open posture, steady voice and facial expression.

The goals of one individual

Keith is a problem drinker and has difficulty asserting himself when he is with his friends. In particular, he is unable to say 'no' when pressed to have an alcoholic drink. One of Keith's goals is to say 'no' confidently, politely and without wavering, in response to group pressure offered in a pub role play situation.

Case example 3 – Mandy is preparing to join a supportive women's group. With the therapist's help, she sets the following aims and goals for herself to achieve over the 8-week course.

– identify own problem issues
– take risks to disclose feelings at least once in each group
– gain a sense of support, power, sense of belonging
– listen to others and respond sensitively
– feel more confident at the end

CHOOSING THE ACTIVITY

Once group aims are established, this determines the category of group activity and the treatment media. Thus an aim to improve skills guides us to employ work or craft activities, while more socially orientated aims will focus us on leisure pursuits or some form of creative therapy. A psychotherapy aim will bias the group towards the creative therapies or simply to have a 'talking' group without activity. Having established the broad category, the next step is to select the specific activity.

Our choice of activity is primarily shaped and constrained both by what individual members will find meaningful and by practical constraints of the environment. Other factors which can influence our choice of the type and level of activity include: the functional level of the members, the mix of members, their level of cohesiveness, and finally, the setting. Each of these will be discussed in turn.

First and foremost, we select our activities through recognizing what will be **meaningful** to the people concerned. Our patients and clients need to have some interest in the group activity, otherwise why should they become involved? The activity should fit the values and beliefs of the individual. If an individual believes art to be childish and demeaning, should this not be respected? Should every housewife be expected to be motivated to join a domestic activity group? Linked to values is the huge area of cultural and religious background which is likely to be a powerful influence on the range of activities a person will accept or enjoy.

The specific activity selected will often be determined by

practical considerations of the **resources and environment**. In work assessment, for example, the activities offered may be limited to clerical, printing and woodwork groups. Although this choice will fit the actual jobs of few of our patients and clients, we can use the principles underlying 'work', and apply these therapeutically to activities we are able to offer.

· In many occupational therapy settings, the type of activity offered is predetermined and choice is limited. Often there is a set departmental structure, for instance, holding a music group on Thursday mornings. Alternatively, departments may be organized to reflect the needs of a particular patient or client population served, for example, doing 'home management' as part of a rehabilitation unit programme. Finally, the choice of groups on offer will be constrained by the skills and inclination of the staff involved. These existing needs may preclude more creative arrangements.

The danger of fixed activity arrangements is that patients and

---

THEORY INTO PRACTICE

Balancing fixed activity programmes with choice

If a department is forced to provide a structured group activity programme, it can maintain a positive edge in three ways. First, the department should provide a variety of types of groups and activities to suit different individuals. The range might include solitary, social work and leisure aspects. It may not be possible to provide the particular activity of interest to a patient or client, but there should be enough choice for any individual to be able to select something consistent with his or her values. Second, groups which operate at different levels should be available. A useful selection would offer groups with a practical bias, groups involving greater emotional intensity and other groups requiring intellectual skills. Third, the programme of group activities available should change as staff, patients or clients move on. The groups offered should be led by need not availability, demand not supply, whenever possible.

clients are simply slotted into an existing structure, rather than having a programme of group activities which are specifically designed for each individual. Ultimately, a balance must be found between what suits individual's needs and what is practical in the context of limited resources.

Often, the choice of the activity itself is secondary to how it is used and experienced by the group. An art activity may be employed within a social, creative or psychotherapy group. These groups offer the same broad activity, but the activity is qualitatively different in terms of its level, demands and what is actually carried out. Four key considerations which influence this aspect of our planning in this way are: the level of the patient or client's functioning, the mix of group members, the level of trust and cohesion and the setting of the group (see Figure 4.7).

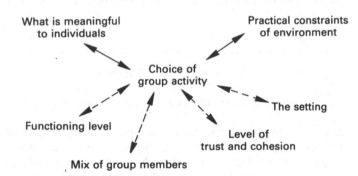

Figure 4.7 Factors influencing choice of group activity.

The functioning level of our group members is a prime consideration. Have the prospective members any particular physical limitations, for instance, mobility problems or being hard of hearing? Are they in an acute phase of a psychiatric illness where we need to take into account the likelihood of members being both vulnerable and unpredictable? What is their level of group skills – their ability to interact and be aware of others' needs? How able are the potential members to focus on the task at hand? What level of stimulation and direction is required? The answers to these questions will critically influence the type, choice and level of group activity offered.

Kaplan (1988) argues that the concept of **optimal arousal level** provides a valuable guide for selecting the level of activity. She suggests that we match an individual's functioning with the demand from the environment. The environment needs to be optimally arousing for patients or clients to encourage them to be energized and alert whilst feeling a little anxious, so challenged. The balance we seek is one where the activity is not too taxing (where the group will become anxious) and also not too under-stimulating (where the group will be bored). In both these extremes, the group members will perform poorly, will be distracted, or will want to leave. Kaplan illustrates this concept by using the following graph (see Figure 4.8).

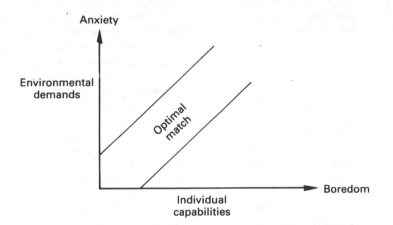

Figure 4.8 Optimal arousal level.

In order to find this optimal match we need to analyse the patient's or client's level of capabilities (namely cognitive capacities, communication skills, emotional needs and perceptual motor skills) and environmental demands (of activities, amount of therapist support and expectations and the degree of group involvement).

The **mix of patients or clients** in the group requires attention, as it can mean the success or failure of a group activity. Are there particular people who do not get on with each other?

THEORY INTO PRACTICE

Optimal arousal level: matching functioning with activity

Functioning level	Capabilities matched to activity
1. Cognitive capacities – limited abstract thought; only able to follow one or two step instructions	Concrete activity chosen; activity is broken down into small steps which are presented in turn <u>Arousal</u>: by offering some more complex instructions
2. Communication skills – most interaction with therapist; minimal contact with others	Craft work to be done on individual basis all around a large table (parallel group level); therapist to encourage interaction between pairs. <u>Arousal</u>: by therapist asking group questions
3. Emotional needs – therapist is significant, guiding person; some vulnerable members easily overwhelmed by others; limited self-awareness	Therapist highly active: meeting needs, supporting, encouraging members; activity is emotionally neutral and does not require self-awareness. <u>Arousal</u>: by encouraging group interaction
4. Perceptual–motor skills – varying degrees of fine motor skill and figure ground perception	Craft work which demands only basic dexterity. <u>Arousal</u>: by encouraging more accurate performance

---

Likewise, are there members who will encourage and support each other? Is the group likely to be so heterogeneous that the group members will find it difficult to relate to each other or will the differences act as a positive force? How helpful is it to have members of the same functioning level together?

The **level of trust and cohesiveness** existing in a group will predetermine the depth of member involvement possible. In a low cohesion group, extra efforts will need to be made to build trust and help members to interact more with each other. Activities which involve personal disclosure or exposure will not be suitable until some trust is established.

Finally, the **actual setting** of the group can have a strong impact, so needs to be considered when planning a group. If it is held in a ward day room, for instance, the group activity may be routinely interrupted or disturbed by events outside the group. Another pertinent illustration is the impact of having a community-based rather than a hospital setting where the issues for, and expectations of members, will be markedly different.

THEORY INTO PRACTICE

Factors influencing choice and level of an art activity group

Note how the choice and level of an art activity changes dramatically once we consider different factors.

Situation 1
patient/client functioning = low
mix of patients/clients = heterogeneous
cohesiveness/trust = lower
setting = ward

Art activity group of choice is to run a **basic activity session** offering a range of techniques. Individuals to work alongside each other on their own projects. Interaction is likely to be limited between members and will be mostly through the therapist.

Situation 2
patient/client functioning = high
mix of patients/clients = homogeneous
cohesiveness/trust = higher
setting = psychotherapy unit

Art activity of choice is a **projective art group**. Session to be structured aiming for in-depth group sharing. Therapist will facilitate but aim for a high level of group involvement.

STRUCTURING THE SESSION

Having made the choice of the type and level of activity, the next step involves creating and planning the full session. In order to do this we can consider the overall structure of the group session in terms of six different phases. These phases differ in quality and emphasis depending upon the type and level of group, but each phase needs to be considered to some degree.

1. **Orientation**. The first phase of any group is the orientation period where it is important to acknowledge each individual and help them feel more at ease. Members should be welcomed individually. A group member, particularly if new, might welcome being offered a seat or cup of tea. Having clues to the activity of the day around (for instance, paints on the table or more explicitly, setting out the aim of the session in writing on a board) can help members adjust from being outside the group to being in the group.

2. **Introduction**. The introduction phase follows soon after and may involve two introductions: a) the members should be introduced to each other if necessary. Simple introductions or a review of people's names may suffice. Some groups may benefit from ice-breaking games such as throwing a bean bag and calling out each other's names. b) The group activity may need some initial explanation. The whole introduction phase may last anything from 30 seconds to 20 minutes depending on the familiarity of the members with each other and the group activity.

3. **Warm-up**. The warm-up phase overlaps with the introduction and similarly varies in time according to how much is needed. Logically, longer warm-up periods are required for new or 'feelings-based' groups. A familiar craft activity group may not require much warm-up space. Typical warm-ups occupational therapists use include: physical exercise to energize a group; humorous activities to relax members; time to look at recipe cards for cooking ideas; verbal games to warm up for a discussion; mime games to prepare for doing role-play.

4. **Action**. This phase is the main part of the session where the activity or activities selected to achieve the group aims are implemented. The action may involve carrying out one task

(for example, baking a cake) or working through a series of exercises (such as in drama therapy). It may be useful to focus on some theme if you have several exercises so that an idea or experience can be followed through.

5. **Wind-down**. Having a period to wind down is important for any group and may be fulfilled in different ways. A closure activity may be used to draw threads together or relax the group. Alternatively, clearing up may signal a transition period towards ending the group. Some psychotherapy groups might rely on the presence of a clock to

---

THEORY INTO PRACTICE

A therapist's plan of an introductory projective art group

1. **Orientation** – welcome members and offer tea as they arrive.
2. **Introduction** – (approximately 10 minutes): a) introduce self, then ask each person to say their names, b) acknowledge newness of group/activity to all members, c) establish aim of not trying to paint 'pretty' pictures but to express self and gain support, d) describe typical format of painting then talking about picture, e) ground rule laid down of no interpretation of paintings except by the individual.
3. **Warm-up** – (approximately 6 minutes): painting to music consisting of different moods and tempos. Aim to have fun, relax group, introduce notion of expressing self through painting. Brief feedback comments at end.
4. **Action** – paint: a) 'how I see myself – what is important to me in my present life', b) 'how I would like it to be'. Each painting to take approximately 15 minutes including sharing and discussion time.
5. **Wind-down** – a) group picture (approximately 5 minutes) using a large piece of paper, start by having a painting conversation with a neighbour, gradually try to have contact with other group members, b) feedback about the group, c) each member invited to say 'one thing positive for me in today's session'.
6. **Post group** – approximately half an hour to write notes and feedback group to team.

allow members to prepare themselves when the time is coming to a close. At the very end of the group, the therapist might conclude with a few key comments and will probably acknowledge each individual by saying 'good-bye'.

6. **Post-group**. It is essential for the leader or leaders to have some time to reflect on the group and record what happened. Leaders may discuss the group, the individuals involved, their roles and may consider future action. For a fuller analysis of this phase, see the section on evaluation in Chapter 8.

THE ENVIRONMENT

When we plan a group, we need to pay as much attention to organizing the environment as we do to devising the group activity. This involves attending to concrete, practical aspects which ensure we are sufficiently prepared for a group. It also involves more abstract considerations where the environment is itself the medium through which we communicate what is expected (or not) and our regard for group members. Both of these aspects are explored more fully in this section.

Practical aspects

Practical planning is largely common sense and should take into account furniture, equipment and physical safety. With regard to **furniture**, we might ask the following questions. Do we need chairs and tables or would cushions be preferable? How should the furniture be positioned? Should separate work tables be used to separate members of different functioning levels? These are important decisions, as they have practical implications and they can affect expectations and subsequent interactions.

Equipment and materials needed should be planned in advance and we should ensure that they are in adequate working condition. A games session, for example, may require a long list of equipment including bats, balls, scorecards, prizes, and even protective clothing.

A particular question often raised about equipment is the use of **recording devices**. Considering the use of this one piece of equipment demonstrates just how complicated the planning process can be. If a video camera is to be used in the group session, have the members agreed to be filmed (and ideally signed a consent form)? Will there be the necessary opportunity to discuss the procedure with the group? Is the equipment safe in the room? How much does it impinge on the group and so affect interaction, and how will this be dealt with? Does the relevant person know how to operate the equipment? What will happen to the video-tape after the event? If you can answer these questions satisfactorily you are ready to use such equipment in the group.

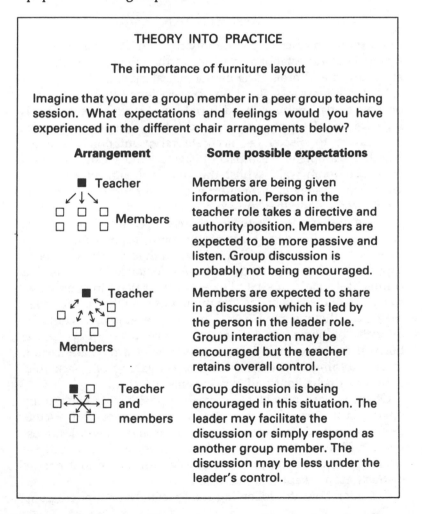

THEORY INTO PRACTICE

The importance of furniture layout

Imagine that you are a group member in a peer group teaching session. What expectations and feelings would you have experienced in the different chair arrangements below?

Arrangement	Some possible expectations
■ Teacher □ □ □ Members □ □ □	Members are being given information. Person in the teacher role takes a directive and authority position. Members are expected to be more passive and listen. Group discussion is probably not being encouraged.
■ Teacher □ □ □ □ □ □ Members	Members are expected to share in a discussion which is led by the person in the leader role. Group interaction may be encouraged but the teacher retains overall control.
■ □ Teacher □ □ and □ □ members	Group discussion is being encouraged in this situation. The leader may facilitate the discussion or simply respond as another group member. The discussion may be less under the leader's control.

We must always promote **physical safety** – namely comply with Health and Safety regulations and consider the safe handling of materials, equipment and substances. We also need to check whether or not there is adequate light, warmth, ventilation and space for comfort. Whilst these latter aspects may not be totally in our control, we should be aware of their potential positive and negative effects on the group. An energetic game of 'tag' for instance, may not be the best choice in a room that is already warm and contains obstacles.

Abstract aspects

On a more abstract level, the environment can communicate much about expectations and can set the scene by creating an atmosphere and promoting emotional safety.

Powerful messages about our **expectations** can be implicit in our choice of equipment and furniture. An example of this is how we might supply only thick paint brushes in a projective art session to discourage accurate representation paintings. Another example is the impact of having good artistic paintings on an art room wall. Whilst this makes for an attractive environment, it may also threaten potential group members who see it as signalling they are expected to be artistic.

When we try to create an **atmosphere**, we first need to consider whether or not our group room has any other functions and associations which might impinge on the members' experience. A group of children, for instance, might find it confusing to suddenly be allowed to 'free play' in their classroom, or alternatively, be taught maths in what is normally their play therapy room. As a different example, it could be difficult for some out-patients to return to a group in the hospital as this carries painful memories of a past admission, to say nothing of the possibility of provoking old 'sick role' patterns of behaviour and expectations.

Often, we can take steps to create a positive atmosphere by offering a nurturing touch, such as providing tea and biscuits to end a group. Similarly, in order to promote a work atmosphere and allow the group to focus on the task at hand, we would lay out the room in a work-like formation and ensure distractions are kept to a minimum.

Consider how the following may facilitate or hinder group

involvement: a) Pop music in the background – this may help to create a relaxed, friendly atmosphere, but if played too loudly, may distract or threaten some people. b) Allowing outside people to drop into a workshop area casually – this may give off a friendly, busy message; equally, it may be distracting and make the workers feel self conscious and exposed in too public an arena. c) Working in a newly built, designer kitchen – for some people, the kitchen may feel uncomfortable and an unfamiliar experience; often, though, having new decorations or furniture helps people feel they are being attended to and valued.

The final aspect of planning the environment involves promoting **emotional safety**. Having a room which is private and free from interruptions is fundamental to any group where feelings are being expressed and building trust is a key aim. Often, closing the group room door is the signal to begin the group. Sometimes, a separate room is not a practical possibility. In this case, other ways to establish boundaries, such as dividers, might be used.

Preparing the environment is a crucial aspect of planning a

THEORY INTO PRACTICE

Checklist for planning the environment

Concrete aspects:

furniture	– what is needed? how should it be positioned?
equipment	– what is needed? check quantity and quality
physical safety	– check equipment and space check comfort

Abstract aspects:

expectations	– communicated through room, location, furniture, equipment
atmosphere	– any associations? what atmosphere is desired?
emotional safety	– consider privacy consider boundaries

group, but it is not the overriding factor. Often our seating is less than ideal. We may not have an attractive, private space at our disposal, and we may not have the most appropriate equipment and furniture. Such factors should not prevent us from going ahead with our group, as the people in the environment are much more significant than the setting. An enthusiastic group spirit can do much to overcome a dowdy dark room, whereas a bright room does not of itself ensure group spirit!

GRADING AND ADAPTING TREATMENT

The fundamental processes underlying occupational therapy intervention is our capacity to grade and adapt activities in ways which transform 'occupation' into 'therapy'. Though these terms 'grading' and 'adapting' are often used interchangeably, this is an unfortunate practice, as each has its own value in therapy. We systematically **grade** the demands of an activity and the amount of stimulation or pressure within the environment. (If using woodwork, for example, we might plan to increase the length of time a person is expected to work.) We **adapt** an activity to suit the background, ability and values of an individual and the circumstances within a situation. (One example of this is how, on finding out a group member is a vegetarian, we might rearrange a planned chicken lunch cookery session and make a vegetable lasagne instead.) The process of grading focuses on the treatment goals, whilst adapting takes into account the situation or individual's needs.

In this section, I will first explore how to grade activities and then offer some ideas about why and how we adapt treatment.

Grading treatment

Group treatment can be graded in at least five ways, as the examples below demonstrate.

Firstly, the **level of difficulty** of the activity may be gradually increased. One good example of this is in a drama therapy group where the members are slowly introduced to physical contact. Early on in the drama course, the group might play a game of 'hug tag' which allows physical contact to occur in a fun, spontaneous way. The group is later introduced __ trust exercises where members are expected to be sensitive to sensations and others' needs. Towards the end of the course, the members experience a group massage relatively unselfconsciously. The therapist of this group has graded the amount and quality of touch towards promoting group trust and sharing.

Secondly, the activity can be broken down into **component parts** which the patients or clients master step by step. One illustration is provided by the client who aims to work on her difficulties of handling social situations. She joins a photography group consisting of eight people and is initially given a task to sort out negatives with one other client with whom she feels safe. She progresses to working in the dark room with different individuals in turn. Later, as she feels more comfortable, she goes out in a group of four people to take some photographs. She is increasingly encouraged to join into the regular end-of-session whole group discussion.

A third way of grading arises when individuals in a group may have their own **specially graded programmes**. For instance, in a group for people who have sustained head injuries who work twice a week in a market garden, one member's goal is to build up her standing tolerance. Increasingly, she stands rather than sits in the greenhouse whilst potting seeds. For another member, physical tolerance is increased by spending more time digging and planting in the vegetable plot. A third member, as part of a wider cognitive development and work training programme, takes increasing responsibility for stock control and accounts.

A fourth way of grading is to gradually **increase the type and number of roles** people are expected to take within a group. One illustration of this is the formal system of promotion which can occur within therapeutic communities. In one community, for example, members of the baking group provided tea and snacks for the rest of the community. Four residents get elected into committee posts of chair, cookery organizer, treasurer and supplies officer. The other group members 'learn the trade' as workers. When a committee member leaves the unit, the committee roles are re-shuffled and a worker is promoted. In this way most of the members have the opportunity to try out more demanding group roles.

A final case arises where a department may have a **series of groups** that operate at different levels. These can be used within graded programmes as individuals are programmed to progress through set groups. Occupational therapy departments are commonly structured along developmental lines to accommodate people who function at lower and higher skill levels. A department may employ Mosey's (1986) adaptive skills theory and have individuals progress through a sequence of parallel, project and cooperative level groups.

THEORY INTO PRACTICE

Case example of grading amount of support and stress experienced

Ruth is emotionally vulnerable, socially anxious and finds contact with men difficult. Her treatment programme is graded to slowly reduce the staff support offered and increase the stress she has to face.

Early stage: Women's discussion group; staff adopt a gentle, nurturing approach.
Middle stage: Photography group consisting of both men and women; interaction encouraged.
Late stage: Social skills group of men and women; emotionally demanding role plays included.

Adapting treatment

What happens when our well planned session which is designed to apply relevant activity doesn't work in practice or is disrupted by some unexpected event? This is an all too common occurrence as we all know! Clearly, we need to have a contingency plan worked out in advance, about how to adapt the activity if it becomes necessary. As Kaplan (1988, p 83) advises, the best protection to deal with surprises of the group being different from expected, is 'to be comfortable with the process of adapting activities'.

Four common reasons why we might need to adapt a session are:

i) **To allow for different levels of skill, experience, motivation and involvement.** In any one group we may have a wide range of functioning levels which need to be taken into account. One pertinent example is where members vary in terms of their physical capacity and further adaptations are needed for people in wheelchairs.

ii) **To cope with unexpected events.** There are many examples of this such as: a new member arrives without warning; the mood of the group suddenly changes to become over-excited or, perhaps, angry; an individual's project 'fails' and a quick, successful end-product is needed; someone refuses to do a particular activity.

iii) **To offer choice.** Whilst we would not wish to overwhelm a patient or client with too many choices or give the impression we have not prepared anything, it is important to offer a degree of choice. Encouraging individuals to make their own selections gives off messages of 'I respect your decision making; I want you to be active and take some responsibility for what you do'.

iv) **To better meet the values and socio-cultural background of individuals.** Consider how far we recognize and attend to the needs of people who belong to an ethnic minority. Prior to a group we should check if there are any particular religious or cultural taboos which are relevant to the activity; for instance, a group may be due to make Christmas party decorations and one member may be a Jehovah's Witness.

When we adapt treatment, we manipulate two variables : the activity and our role. Of **the activity** we need to ask: does this activity need to be more or less structured? What new balance of fun or emotional intensity is required? Does the activity demand enough or too much of the members? How can it be changed and made more (or less) challenging?

Kaplan (1988, p 88) recommends that we adapt our activities to meet the changing needs of individuals and the group for 'complexity, novelty and uncertainty'. **Complexity** concerns the amount of skill the activity demands. The number of directions given at any one time, the length of time needed and the type of concepts involved are all relevant factors to take into account. If members appear unable to perform or are overwhelmed, the task needs to be broken down into smaller or simpler units. **Novelty** considers the familiarity or newness of an activity. If members seem bored by the same activity, an injection of creativity is required to change it. **Uncertainty** refers to the element of predictability and chance. If no-one understands the rules of a game anxiety will rise; if the game is too obvious, it will be boring. The level that is comfortable for each of these three factors will differ from group to group.

It is no easy task to respond appropriately to each individual within the group situation, as this often means juggling a range of group roles. However, the way we adapt **our approach** is probably more crucial to the therapy than our use of activity.

THEORY INTO PRACTICE

Five tips on how to adapt activities

1. Always have a selection of activities at hand. If, for example, finger painting is the day's activity, have some paint brushes available for those who dislike messing their hands.
2. For a craft type activity, have products available at different stages of completion to offer to those who are unable to concentrate for the full period. In woodwork, you might have a finished article at hand which simply involves varnishing for a quick end-product, one which needs to be assembled and one which has to be made from scratch.
3. Have several alternatives planned to cope with changes in tempo or mood. For example, an aggressive, over-stimulated group will benefit more from a quietening, relaxing wind-down activity than a fun, lively one. Similarly, plan to do role plays in pairs if some members feel too threatened to act in front of the group.
4. Research the social, cultural and religious background of the group members. How strongly do they adhere to their practices? What are the implications for activities?
5. Never be rigid with your plan of action. It is easy at times to have a strong belief or investment in a particular activity, but if it is not working we need to be able to 'let it go'.

We can adapt our role in three main ways: first, we might modify the **amount of support** we offer, or consider the differing degrees to which we nurture individuals or protect them from failure. Second, our **expectations** might be modified, for instance by demanding different standards of performance. Third, we can adapt the **amount of direction** and instruction we give, depending on members abilities and the familiarity of the situation.

MOTIVATING GROUP MEMBERS

Last but not least on our planning agenda, we need to consider how to gain (and retain) our group members. (Referral procedures and advertising issues are discussed in the following chapter.) The question of how we motivate individuals to join a group is the specific issue addressed in this section.

One dilemma that continually confronts us is what to do with patients and clients who are reluctant to join an activity or group. How should we respond? Should we respect their wishes? Is it acceptable to try persuasion tactics? What is the best way to encourage someone? I will attempt to answer these questions by exploring some of the underlying dynamics about what may be happening when someone is reluctant to come to a group. The answer to the question of what to do as a therapist follows naturally from this understanding. Different strategies for encouraging individuals to attend a group will then be discussed and evaluated.

The reluctant attender

The reasons why a person may be reluctant to attend a group are many and complex. Five different scenarios are offered below, together with some ideas about how then to handle the situation.

1. The individual feels the occupational therapy group will **not be beneficial or relevant**. Alternatively, he or she is not motivated to work on problem areas.

   There may be some room for discussion in this case, particularly about the aims and benefits of the group. A 'try-it-you-might-like-it' approach may work. Ultimately, however, we must respect a person's choice. Indeed, the person's non-compliance can be viewed as a healthy sign. Our patients and clients will often be right about what they will find beneficial – who are we to argue the point?

2. An individual is **ignorant or feels confused** about what the group offers. This is often signalled by questions such as, 'Do I have to come?' or comments such as 'I don't want to make a basket again, thank you'.

   Clear but gentle explanation is the response frequently required in this situation. As in the previous scenario, answers should be given about how the group might help the individual. He or she may find it useful to speak with other group members to get their (hopefully positive!) viewpoint.

3. The person **lacks drive and feels apathetic and disinterested**. Patients or clients who are institutionalized or who have chronic mental illnesses commonly experience these feelings. Apathy may also be a product of the person's condition or illness, or be a side effect of medication.

   In this case, it is crucial to find a 'motivator' – something which will increase the meaningfulness of the activity for the person. We might employ external reinforcement, for example use a token economy approach. Equally, we could appeal to the person's own interests, skills and values, for instance, by offering a practical end-product. It is also important to offer choices and include the person in the planning process as this will help to increase his or her investment in the group. An example here is getting individuals to negotiate about where they are to go on a camping trip. The members who take part in the decision are much more likely to be more committed to the plan than a person who is given no such choice.

4. The prospective group member is reluctant to come to the group because he or she is **anxious, worried, suspicious or simply unsure of** what to expect. These sorts of feelings may manifest in comments like 'I'm not very good at talking in groups' or 'What will you expect me to do?'

   Reassurance in the form of 'It will be all right – nothing to worry about' is not a helpful response to someone who is expressing anxieties. Coming out with such platitudes usually means we are not taking seriously fears that deserve to be acknowledged. We may be comfortable and experienced in groups ourselves and have forgotten how terrifying it can be for the novice. So, we need to work on alleviating the fears by listening, understanding and then reassuring where appropriate. We should explore the person's reservations about joining, and then ideally, make a joint decision about whether or not the group could be a positive experience. Inviting the person to talk to someone else in the group whom he or she trusts, can also help. Alternatively, a compromise might be effective where the reluctant person just comes to observe and meet the group members – a simple form of desensitization.

5. A person is unwilling to join a group because of **external factors** such as wider group dynamics. The individual may be modelling on other patients or clients who are refusing treatment. Alternatively, he or she may be having some problem with or trying to avoid another member of the group. Also, we should recognize (with regret) that it may be other staff who are deliberately or unconsciously sabotaging the group.

   If dynamics like these seem to apply, it is crucial to try to understand exactly what is happening. Is it a problem which needs to be tackled head on? What is the individual gaining by not joining the group? If there are staff 'sabotage' dynamics around, issues of competition or angry feelings may be relevant. Efforts should be made to sort this out directly, through negotiation or confrontation, rather than act it out through a confused patient or client.

Encouraging attendance

There are several strategies we can use to motivate individuals to join a group – some positive and some negative.

The **positive strategies** we can try include:

a) **Persuasion by explanation** – the person needs to know why and how he or she may be involved and that there is a meaningful goal to work towards. Natural fears and false expectations can be explored.

b) **Negotiated contract** – this can be formally written up or simply spoken. The terms of joining the group should be clear, including what the individual may gain by attending and what can be realistically expected from it. The therapist might offer something in return (for instance some one-to-one time).

c) **Preparatory interview** – often a two-way clarification of needs and expectations is useful. The patient or client can share aspects he or she wants to work on or the therapist might explain how the group could help. This interview could be followed up by an introduction to the group, room or relevant members.

d) **Involvement in planning.** The patient or client as mentioned before, could have some involvement in the planning of the group to increase his or her investment in it. At the very least, the prospective member should be given choice as to what type of group he or she would find most interesting or useful.

Two **negative strategies** which are sometimes rather unthinkingly applied are deception or coercion. We occasionally fall into the trap of practising **deceptions** such as inviting a patient or client to join a social activity or 'come for a chat', when privately, we have a more therapeutic purpose in mind. It is tempting to place the importance on getting the patient or client into the group and then he or she will benefit. In fact, this strategy of the end justifying the means is counter-productive as the deception cannot be maintained and the trust will eventually be broken. More fundamentally, it goes against the occupational therapy philosophy of encouraging cooperative treatment planning.

A more pernicious practice is the use of **coercion**. This is most overt when patients are physically handled and brought into occupational therapy despite their protests – a practice which is professionally and ethically intolerable. Coercion of a more covert type arises in situations where a therapist (or institution) has some power over the patient or client. A number of examples come to mind: a drug abuser who has chosen treatment rather than a prison term may be 'forced' to attend therapy groups; the institutionalized person with a chronic mental illness who is too compliant to take an active stand; the psychiatric in-patient who is forced to attend ward groups under threat of being discharged for not complying with treatment. Ultimately, forcing someone into a group may ensure he or she physically attends but it does not guarantee the person will participate or become usefully engaged in the activity. In fact, it is often counter-productive for the group as a whole, as negativism can be contagious and a person's resentment or apathy may sabotage the rest of the group.

THEORY INTO PRACTICE

The pros and cons of reminding a patient or client to attend OT

Option 1. Giving the patient or client an at-the-time prompt that the group is starting such as ringing up the ward to send 'X' down.
Pros – i) The patient or client may need the small reminder having lost track of time or due to memory difficulties. ii) Ringing the ward includes the nurses in the treatment which ensures a better team approach and reminds them of occupational therapy issues
Cons – i) The patient or client may feel unduly pressured and with the direct prompt may feel unable to refuse. ii) Others may use coercion or stress inappropriate reasons to attend if they have to step in to give the reminder.
Option 2. Giving an advance reminder, for example, 'See you at the group tomorrow'.
Pros – The additional reminder may be helpful and make the patient or client feel more expected or wanted and generate enthusiasm.
Cons – This can often be impractical. We cannot give out reminders all the time with each group member.
Option 3. Once the arrangement has been agreed, leave it to the patient's or clients's own initiative to turn up.
Pros – This method shows respect to the patient or client and allows him or her to take responsibility.
Cons – i) Avoidance of the group may be the easiest way for a patient or client to handle any stress and this approach gives an avoidance opportunity. ii) More dependent or less-able patients or clients may need a prompt.

Overall, deception and coercion are counter-productive if the result is that someone in the group is likely to be negative, resistant or not actively involved. It also jeopardizes the value of the group for others. Attendance should be the result of mutual negotiation, understanding, preparation and involvement.

In summary, preparing for a session necessarily involves a good deal of careful and explicit planning. We need to consider:

- aims and goals
- the activity
- the structure of the session
- the environment
- how to grade and adapt the treatment
- how to motivate members to attend.

Decisions need to be taken for each of these interconnecting points. Whilst the process of planning for a session can seem a bit laborious, to be effective, it should not be rushed. If occupational therapists do not carefully plan their groups, they are in danger of offering activity for its own sake. Therapeutic activity is not accidental. Planning treatment is a challenging exercise in problem-solving and creativity.

5

Planning groups: setting up a group

Setting up a group demands planning, organization, judgement, problem-solving and a willingness to look for creative solutions. This chapter first explains the **sequence** of setting up a group and emphasizes the importance of giving time to preparation and planning. Subsequent sections consider the decisions that need to be made about **membership** and **time factors** of the group and discuss the processes of **gaining referrals** and **preparing members**.

PLANNING SEQUENCE

The process of setting up a group usually involves working through a series of tasks or stages. Depending on the group, the stages will create different problems and assume differing degrees of importance.

The flow chart in Figure 5.1 below presents a common sequence of action when setting up a group.

i)   Initially, there needs to be a **demand** for a group. This may be signalled by patient or client needs or equally may come from an interested staff member.

ii) Decisions about the **type and level** of group are made after considering the wider context (for instance noting groups already in existence) and identifying resources available (namely staff, time, equipment and space). Two main decisions need to be made. One is the membership issue of who should be involved. Then there are the time-factor decisions concerning how long and how often the group should meet.

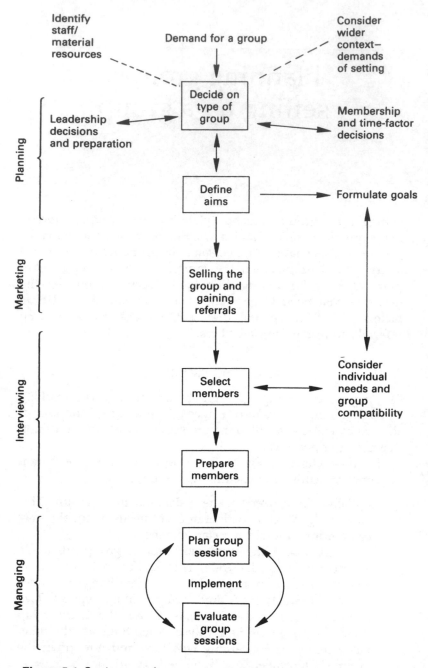

Figure 5.1 Setting up of a group: sequence of action.

iii) Next, the **aims** should be formulated, and if necessary re-formulated in the light of subsequent decisions. Group goals need to be set.

iv) Having carried through the preliminary planning, the next stage is to gain **referrals**. Referral procedures need to be set (such as designing a form) and the group advertised in a way appropriate to the unit (for example using leaflets and letters).

v) **Members are then selected** for the group bearing in mind both their individual needs and issues of compatibility.

vi) The next stage of **preparing the members** and engaging them in the group can be a crucial one as it can make the difference about whether or not the group begins and continues.

vii) Only at this penultimate stage should specific attention be paid to **planning the content** of the sessions in detail. Whilst it is tempting to rush ahead, we cannot come to a final decision about a session until we know the members' needs.

viii) Lastly, constant **evaluation** of the group is necessary and plans are likely to be modified after each session.

The process of setting up and planning a group is often the hardest part of undertaking groupwork. It can seem both lengthy and laborious, while the actual running of the group often seems more exciting and rewarding. However, the planning stage is not only vital to maximizing the chances of ensuring that the group actually works well; it can also be satisfying in its own right. It should be viewed as a creative process where we design a treatment, solve different problems and think through strategies for how to get a group to 'feel' right. It is not simply a question of going through a set sequence in a mechanical fashion. Whittaker (1985, p 12) expresses this nicely when she says, 'working out a suitable structure is an act of the imagination.'

Despite the importance of systematic planning and careful reasoning, we should not be rigidly ruled by our plan. A group and its leader must be free to respond spontaneously. One illustration of this is provided by an occasion when I had planned a dance session for a group of adolescents. On the day, several members were unable to come to the session, leaving only five of us. With so few people, members felt too self conscious to dance and the planned pairwork was impractical. The group members and I agreed a change of plan. We decided to postpone the dance session and enjoyed a quiet music appreciation group instead.

MEMBERSHIP DECISIONS

Three decisions need to be made about the membership of the group. These concern: a) whether the group should be open or closed; b) the size of group; c) the composition of group members.

Open versus closed groups

Closed groups start and finish with the same group members and will usually run for a fixed number of sessions (for instance a 12 session Anxiety Management Course). This gives time for members to build relationships and trust each other. In contrast, **open groups** allow members to join and leave the group as they wish. A group run on an acute admission ward, for example, may have a completely different membership from week to week. Other open groups may contain a few core members who accommodate newcomers as necessary. Sometimes, it may be possible to run a **semi-open group** where membership is stable over a long period but takes a new member if anyone leaves. Similarly, an open group may be closed for fixed periods but accept new referrals at set times.

The choice of open or closed membership depends on the type of group and members involved. **Support groups** are likely to need a period of stability to allow members to build up trust and feel safe in the group. A closed or semi-open group would encourage the development of these relationships and a group ethos. **Activity groups**, where the focus is on the activity at hand or on individual achievement, can operate as open groups more easily, since newcomers are less likely to be disruptive. Indeed, these groups may benefit from the stimulus provided by changing faces. In terms of members involved, the security of a closed group may be needed for any member who finds groups difficult or is socially anxious. If members are likely to be inconsistent attenders, then an open group is the best option, ideally in combination with a few regulars who act as 'culture carriers'.

The advantages and disadvantages of each type of group are summarized in Table 5.1 below.

Size of group

Ideally, the aims of the group and needs of its members should determine its size. In a **work or task group** where the people require individual attention or teaching, four to six members is usually an ideal size. A **psychotherapy group** usually works best with five to nine members. This is small enough to be intimate, supportive and safe for disclosure, yet large enough

Table 5.1 Advantages and disadvantages of open and closed groups

	Advantages	*Disadvantages*
Open group	more practical for certain settings greater variety of resources available with new members providing stimulation group can operate with fluctuating attendance opportunity to work on issues of change and adaptability	unpredictable membership makes it hard to plan and to target treatment specifically for individuals in advance relationships more superficial with less group cohesion and trust less intimacy, disclosure sub-groups/cliques can form making it difficult for new members to be accepted
Closed group	group can be more specifically planned and targeted deeper relationships occur with greater cohesion and trust depth of content and level of disclosure increased more consistent and predictable, so safer	tendency for group to get 'stuck' with members operating in set roles may not be feasible in certain settings group dependent on members' commitment – may have to fold if several drop out less opportunity to deal with change and adapting to others

to operate as a group. **Social or communication groups**, for example dance or drama groups, might select eight or more members – large enough to give the group 'energy' and allow some members to blend in with the crowd, yet small enough to ensure personal recognition. Less commonly, we may be involved in a **large group** of between 20 and 50 members. This special type of group is mostly seen in the form of community meetings within therapeutic community environments.

To decide how many members to include we need to balance the amount of attention each individual needs with the practical constraints of staff resources and the type of activity. Remembering that the point of using a group is to tap the rich dynamics and support available, the group needs to be large enough to include a diversity or balance of members. Too few members may mean we end up giving a series of individual therapy sessions. On the other hand, the group should be small enough for individuals to feel comfortable (that is to say not socially anxious) but not so small as to increase their self-consciousness.

There are advantages and disadvantages to both small and large groups. The main arguments about group size are laid out in Table 5.2. One point to bear in mind, however, is that

Table 5.2 Advantages and disadvantages of smaller versus larger groups

	Advantages	*Disadvantages*
The smaller the group	easier for members to contribute greater intimacy and depth safer, less threatening and more predictable	group can become 'stuck'; norms and roles too established pressure on members who wish to be more passive less resources and energies to draw
The larger the group	more energy, resources and creativity to draw on diversity of people and experiences may be efficient use of time	less freedom for expression more members under-involved higher numbers can be anxiety provoking and intimidating greater danger of cliques forming

group size is often subjective. A group of ten strangers can feel too large, whilst a cohesive drama group of 20 members can feel intimate.

Composition of group members

As we select members for a group, we need to pay some attention to obtaining the combination of particular individual characteristics which will make for the most effective group. We might note the gender, age or status of individuals, their functioning level or their particular problem areas. To what extent should members be similar to each other, and in what ways?

There are no hard and fast rules about the best composition of members, though three points should be borne in mind. First, we would probably want to avoid any arrangement which unduly isolates one individual, for instance, having one woman in an all male group. Second, members should be able to identify with each other, at least to some extent. The group may not 'gel' if members' problems, concerns or functioning levels are too disparate; for instance, it is inadvisable to mix acutely ill in-patients with more stable out-patients. On the other hand, more heterogeneous groups provide greater opportunities for problem solving as they present us with a wider range of ideas and perspectives offered by different

---

THEORY INTO PRACTICE

Group composition decisions

Consider the following examples of occupational therapy groups and the different decisions made about group composition. Do you agree with the rationales offered?

1. A **woodwork activity session** is planned to include 'novices' and 'experts'. This is accepted as the experts will help the novices, thereby increasing interaction. Individual's aims of treatment (and problems) vary from improving task performance to encouraging hobby interest. The group is a fairly disparate one, though in its own way, it gels.

2. A **men's support group** is planned. Group leaders ensure that all (male) members are motivated and can cope with speaking in such a group. The men's areas of concern vary and span: problems with relationships or work, issues of sexuality and stress concerning the problem of living up to ideal masculine stereotypes.

3. Different people are referred to an **art group** – some to improve task skills and some to encourage emotional expression. The therapist decides to place the members into two separate groups (art versus projective art) as a different style of therapy and activity is required.

4. A treatment team involved in treating people with eating disorders run a **psychotherapy group** for women with the problem of bulimia to share their feelings. The team decide against a similar group for the women with a diagnosis of anorexia nervosa because of the dangers that they may reinforce each other's life threatening behaviour.

5. The staff selecting out-patients for a **leisure group** that offers outings to community facilities, establish the criteria for attendance as: a) lack of overt disturbance b) ability to travel independently c) social isolation where the member does not have other social outlets.

6. A **task group** is formed with members who have long term psychiatric disorders and a low functional level. Group activities involve short-term, concrete projects. The members differ widely in both age and diagnosis.

7. An occupational therapist is asked to run a ward **drama-therapy group**. She leaves the group composition up to individual choice and so increases the likelihood of getting more motivated members.

members. Benson (1987, p 23) succinctly summarizes these ideas by advising that 'groups should be **similar** enough to ensure commonality of need and compatibility but **disparate** enough to ensure that members will be stimulated and useful to each other.'

TIME FACTOR DECISIONS

Four time factor issues need to be addressed when setting up a group: a) the day and time of the group; b) length of session; c) frequency of meetings; d) whether the group should be open-ended or time-limited. Each of these issues is briefly discussed below.

Day and time

A number of considerations come into play when choosing the day and time for a group to run. First, at a practical level, we need to consider the availability of resources (staffing and the room).

Second, we need to take into account the activities or groups our patients or clients attend before and after the group. Consider for example, the impact on an individual of experiencing a counselling session just before a projective art group. The person is likely to feel emotionally tired and reluctant to disclose any more feelings, or alternatively, will be 'warmed up' and come in at a different level to other members.

Third, individuals' natural rhythms may be relevant. Classic examples of this are that elderly people are often more alert in the mornings whilst people suffering from endogenous depression are likely to operate better in the afternoons.

Fourth, we need to consider the practice and programme of the wider unit. In a hospital for instance, it may be advisable not to run groups during ward-round times if patients are likely to be taken out of the group as a result.

Length of the session

The length of time for a session needs to allow opportunity for the group to get going but should take into account members' capacities. Too short a session will result in frustration and unfinished business, and leave people less motivated to become involved next time. On the other hand, too long a session is likely to be boring and too physically or emotionally demanding.

The type of group will often define the time limit. **Support groups** tend to need more time than individual sessions as it takes a group longer to warm up and establish a theme. Yalom (1975) recommends a period of at least 60 minutes for psychotherapy groups (which allows for the unfolding and working through of themes) but less than 2 hours (as there is a point of diminishing returns when the group becomes repetitive).

Activity groups can run from anything between half an hour to all day depending on the particular occupational therapy task being undertaken.

Perhaps more important than the length of allocated time for a group is the fact of having a clearly **set time-limit**. Group members need to know when their group will end. This allows members to pace themselves. Ending at a pre-determined time will also help members to feel safer and more secure in the knowledge that expectations will be met.

Any therapist engaged in emotional work with individuals or groups will recognize that the last 10 minutes of a session often contain the most significant material. You might find a situation towards the end of a group where a member discloses a traumatic incident or begins to express a deep feeling. Whilst it will be tempting to prolong the group in order to work through the emotions – don't (!) or at least **try** to end at the proper time. Ask yourself why the member has made such an important announcement at the end when it cannot be followed up. I would suggest that the material may have been shared precisely **because of** the safety net of the group finishing shortly. The person may not yet be ready for a fuller exploration. If the person is ready, the group can always return to the issue the following session.

Frequency of meetings

The decision of how often to run a group should take into account both the type of group and the needs of its members. A social skills group, for example, may operate best with a fortnightly slot which will allow opportunities to practise and so generalize skills learned, outside the group. A reality orientation session may be offered daily to maintain regular cognitive stimulation. In contrast, a daily group would be inconvenient and unnecessary for higher functioning out-patients.

Whittaker (1985) recommends that we should balance three criteria: intensity, importance and continuity. **Intensity** of experience is increased with more frequent meetings. This may or may not be desirable. The **importance** of the group is seen in the context of the comparative importance of outside life. Too much emphasis on the group may foster a dependence and result in an unnatural focus where group relationships are seen as more important than the 'real' relationships outside. **Continuity** refers to how easily members can make links between sessions. If it is important for one session to feed into another, a twice weekly group may be best, whereas, a group with a different theme each session could occur on a weekly or fortnightly basis. Using this formula, we might aim for continuity and intensity for some groups and meet twice weekly, and aim for continuity and less importance for other groups and meet fortnightly.

Open-ended versus time-limited groups

An open-ended group is one which is intended to continue for an indefinite period of time. Many of our occupational therapy **activity groups** fall into this category. The groups are on offer for the patients' and clients' benefit and only cease with changes of staffing, resources, policy or demand. The main advantage of this system is the continuity it offers – staff and patients or clients will know about, and so use, the service available.

Support groups tend to operate best with a time limit. A social skills training course, for instance, may include 12 sessions, each with a set agenda and objectives. If group members would benefit from further training at the end, another, higher level, group could then be offered. Another example of a time-limited group which makes sense is an anxiety management group where clients learn about anxiety and coping techniques in an organized way. At some point members will have been taught all the relevant techniques and need to go away to apply them.

The advantage of having a fixed number of sessions is that members can pace themselves and make better use of the limited time. Group members are likely to be more focused in their intent to gain from the group in such circumstances.

GAINING REFERRALS

The process of gaining referrals to a newly set up group involves two separate tasks: advertising the group and establishing an appropriate referral system.

Advertising the group

Different groups in their respective settings will demand different levels of 'advertising'. In some situations all we need to do is inform team members of the proposed start date and request referrals. Alternatively, we might adopt a more formal

---

THEORY INTO PRACTICE

Sample of an 'advertising' letter to a GP*

15 October, 1992

Dear Dr Stone,

Re: New Support Group for Women with Physical Disabilities

May I draw your attention to a new support group we are planning to offer in the new year, for women with physical disabilities. The group will take place in this Occupational Therapy Department every Tuesday between 2:00 and 4:00 pm for 12 weeks starting from 12 January, 1993.

The main **aims** of the group are: a) to identify stressful situations in which the women have felt 'disabled', b) To explore ways of dealing with these, c) To promote self confidence by recognizing existing strengths, d) To gain support from the sharing and exchange of experiences.

The **method** of treatment will be discussion-based but will also include the use of activities, video, role play and guest speakers.

We would be pleased to accept any referrals for women you consider might benefit from this group. The closing date for referrals will be 5 December, 1992.

If either you or a prospective group member would like further information, please do not hesitate to contact us on the above telephone number.

Yours sincerely,

Karen Black and Sheila Edwards
Senior Occupational Therapists

(*information based on a referral form designed by Ben McPhillips and Rachael Glennane, East Hill House, Essex Social Services)

---

approach and send out a letter about the group to relevant referring agencies. At other times we might need to employ more active marketing strategies in order to 'sell' the group to prospective consumers or referrers. Whichever advertising strategy is adopted, we should be explicit about the aims of the proposed group, who will benefit and the procedures for referral. View this as an important public relations exercise. Done well, it ensures both suitable referrals for the group and promotes our work as therapists and professionals.

Referral systems

The practice of how patients or clients are referred to a group is diverse as these different options show. 1) Whilst most groups require specific referrals, a few operate on the basis of 'blanket' (unplanned) referrals. 2) Some groups insist that referrals can only come from certain sources (for example doctors) whilst other groups accept from various sources. 3) In terms of procedure, groups may request either written or verbal referrals. This section focuses on these three points of debate about which is the most effective referral system.

Blanket versus planned referrals

Occasionally occupational therapy groups operate blanket referral systems whereby any patient or client can come into whichever group is on offer at the time. It is most commonly seen when therapists are based on a ward and this system ensures he or she has access to all patients without having to wait for official referrals. Blanket referrals may be practical on wards where there is a high turnover of patients or their unstable health means the group membership cannot be predicted from week to week. Members are invited to join on the day if they 'feel up to it'.

Whilst this arrangement may be practical, it has its drawbacks. In the first place, occupational therapists cannot adequately plan a group and gear it to individual's needs. Secondly, when we slot people into an activity without adequate assessment, we are in danger of providing diversion rather than applying treatment. Lastly, we are likely to be confronted with people we do not know and at the very least, this is disconcerting. If we are ignorant of precautions, for example with a violent patient, it can be dangerous.

So, barring exceptional circumstances, we ought to have a planned system whereby we set a ceiling number for a group and then invite relevant referrals. In this way, we can consider, in advance, the suitability of prospective members. Armed with the knowledge of who will attend a group, our treatment planning will be more specific and focused.

Sources of referral

Who should be able to refer to a group is one decision which needs to be made in the context of the unit's accepted practice. This may mean that referrals to an occupational therapy group can only be made by the doctors, by the treatment team, or by the occupational therapists themselves. An alternative possibility is to ask for self-referrals only.

Keeping the occupational therapists in control often ensures appropriate referrals. On the other hand, widening the source of referrals may mean more prospective members and greater treatment team involvement. Self-referrals usually ensure that the prospective member is motivated to join the group. Whichever procedure is adopted, group leaders should ensure that the group aims and criteria for selection of members are clearly communicated. Referrers need to be able to make an informed decision about who best to refer.

Written versus verbal referrals

The choice of whether to accept written or verbal referrals again depends on the accepted practice. However, the current emphasis on documentation and quality assurance suggests that in the absence of a written referral, we should record the details of the verbal request.

This recorded information assists the leader by providing a baseline for treatment and ensures that key data is at hand, rather than having to search out medical notes for instance.

When designing a form, occupational therapists need to be clear about what we need and want to ask. Consider how best to minimize the effort for the referrer – if the form is too unwieldy it will not be used effectively. The content of a form

```
┌─────────────────────────────────────────────────────┐
│              THEORY INTO PRACTICE                    │
│                                                     │
│             A sample referral form                  │
│                                                     │
│  Referral from: _____        Date: _____   │
│                                                     │
│  NAME: _____  DATE OF BIRTH: _____     │
│                                                     │
│  ADDRESS: _____ │
│  _____│
│                                                     │
│  GROUP REQUESTED: _____ │
│  REASON FOR REFERRAL: _____ │
│  _____│
│  _____│
│  _____│
│                                                     │
│  SPECIAL CONSIDERATIONS (e.g. precautions, special  │
│  needs, level of cooperation expected):             │
│  _____│
│  _____│
│                                                     │
│  Signed: _____        Date: _____  │
└─────────────────────────────────────────────────────┘
```

might include: the facts about the prospective member; date of referral and who it is from; reason for referral; and any precautions.

PREPARING PROSPECTIVE MEMBERS

The preparation of prospective members for a group is a crucial process as the group's effectiveness depends on members being 'engaged' and prepared to function in the group. Usually this preparation will take the form of a one-to-one pre-group interview, although occasionally a quick informal chat will suffice. It is an opportunity both for prospective member and leader to meet, and for us to assess in advance, the potential usefulness of the group for the individual. The time can be used to build mutual trust and understanding and is a two-way process of giving and gaining information.

Some preparation is essential as members will have questions about the group, and leaders will want to establish time, dates and a mutual commitment to the treatment. At a deeper level, members will often feel ambivalent about joining a group, uncertain about its nature and purpose and anxious about what will be demanded of them. This uncertainty or stress about the group can create defensive or hostile barriers and result in passive or aggressive behaviour – behaviours that are usually unhelpful to both the person and the group.

The pre-group interview

The pre-group interview has multiple aims:

1. **To introduce** the prospective member and therapist to each other – when the group starts, the patient or client will recognize at least one familiar face. For the therapists, it is a useful opportunity to build an impression of how best to approach the individual.
2. **To give information** about the group – the therapist will describe the nature and purpose of the group and explain any practical details as relevant. An outline of what can be expected in the first or a typical session is usually helpful. This also allows the prospective member an opportunity to ask questions and express any concerns.
3. **To provide a baseline assessment** of problem areas – this is particularly relevant for groups with clearly defined objectives. A self-rating questionnaire may be given to the individual, for instance, in order to establish weekly goals for a social skills group. The assessment can then be applied at the end of the group to evaluate progress.
4. **To negotiate aims and goals** – it is important to bring together the individual's and group's aims or goals. This process of clarifying aims of treatment is central to each member's motivation.
5. **To clarify member's expectations** – the individual may have unrealistic aims for the group or misconceptions about its purpose or method. These will then need to be re-negotiated.
6. **To acknowledge reservations and anxieties** about the group – the interview is an opportunity for the member to ask

questions and express feelings. Members may need reassurance that, for example, they will not be forced to do anything against their will and that others will be in a similar position.

7. **To establish ground rules and group rules** – a contract of attendance (written or verbal) may be negotiated, stating how many sessions can be missed or the need to participate actively. This should be a two-way process of shared responsibility, with the leader enquiring in turn what the member would like from him or her.

THEORY INTO PRACTICE

An example contract

Susan Ashe is a patient in a work assessment programme who has long-standing behavioural difficulties. A formal, written contract is negotiated to help her keep involved in the group treatment:

Contract for attending the occupational therapy clerical group

I, Susan Ashe, agree to:

1. attend the clerical group every Monday and Thursday for the next 4 weeks to practise my clerical skills and working with others.
2. stay for at least half an hour.
3. carry out clerical activities of my choice.
4. not break this contract. If I do, I understand this group will no longer be open to me.

Signed _____   Date _____

I, Karen Toby, Occupational Therapist, agree to:

1. offer the facilities of the clerical group to Susan Ashe, in order that she may practise her clerical and social skills.
2. the negotiated conditions of Susan attending for at least half and hour and choosing her own tasks.
3. offer plenty of encouragement.

Signed _____   Date _____

8. **To begin to build a relationship** of mutual trust and respect – by taking time to discuss the group with the prospective member, the therapist signals that the group is a collaborative venture and not a treatment to be imposed on passive individuals.

Yalom (1975) recommends the following procedure for preparation. (Although he is referring to preparation for a psychotherapy group, note the relevance for other types of groups also.) i) Patients are presented with a brief explanation of group psychotherapy. ii) Patients are advised to be honest and direct about their feelings in the here and now though reassured it will not be a forced confessional. iii) Patients are forewarned about feeling puzzled or discouraged about the group's benefit in early meetings, but are urged to stay with the group. They are also told that many find it difficult to disclose their feelings. iv) The historical development of group therapy and some research about its benefits are then described to instil faith in its method. v) Confidentiality is discussed along with issues of extra-group socializing (not recommended).

Yalom and his colleagues (1967) tested the effectiveness of such preparation in a controlled experiment on 60 patients going on to group therapy. Half were seen in a 30 minute preparatory session, whilst the others were seen for an equal period of time in a conventional history taking interview. Later, the prepared members were found to have more faith in therapy (which in turn positively influenced outcomes) and engaged in more interaction than the non-prepared.

In conclusion, this chapter has described the stages of preparation necessary in order to set up a longer term group. First, decisions need to be made about the membership of the group – namely its size, composition and whether it is to be open or closed. Then, time factor decisions concerning how long and how often the group should run need to be made. After that, the group is ready to be advertised and an appropriate referral system needs to be created. Finally, prospective members need to be prepared for the group.

The process of setting up a group can be time-consuming but each stage of planning is important for ensuring the success of the overall programme. Once planning is completed, the group is ready to begin – an exciting, if somewhat nerve-racking time for prospective group leaders. The next four chapters explore different aspects of the leader's involvement once a group is up and running.

6

Leadership

The success of any therapy group depends largely on the effectiveness of the leader. Chapters 4 and 5 stressed that an important part of that effectiveness depends on occupational therapists planning, thinking through and organizing well. But that is not the whole story – we have to **run** the group effectively, too!

When running a group we aim to create a positive environment in which people can grow and learn. To this end, we need to set the pace, level and content of the activities, and to guide members' participation. In the course of a session we may adopt a myriad of roles, respond to changing demands and solve numerous problems as they arise. These are complex processes – no simple formula can hope to explain how to lead, let alone how to be a good leader. We may be fortunate in that some of the skills needed may occur naturally within us. Many of the skills can be learned regardless of natural gifts. However, it is also important to recognize our limitations. There will always be some kind of groupwork which we are not equipped to handle and we need to acknowledge this to ourselves and to others.

Given these constraints, the first step to becoming an effective leader is to appreciate the impact our behaviour can have on a group and in turn, the effect the group can have on ourselves as leader. We are then in a position to evaluate how best to adapt our role to meet the differing demands of each group and can ask questions such as: What degree of responsibility should I, as leader, assume? Would the group benefit from my adopting a directive or non-directive approach? Are two leaders preferable to one? If so, how should we work together? This chapter offers an opportunity to reflect on three separate issues involved with the leadership of a group. The first section considers the **role** of the leader. The second considers leadership **style** and how this both shapes and is shaped by, the group. The final section discusses the issue of **co-leadership**, its advantages and disadvantages, and how to make the partnership work. Whilst much of the content is applicable to any group, my specific focus is leadership within therapy groups.

THE LEADER ROLE

This section tries to unravel some of the complexities of the role of leader. It first explores these roles and functions of a leader in the context of an occupational therapy group. Then the roles specific to activity and support groups are examined in turn. Roles also carry with them certain responsibilities and these are discussed in the final section.

Role functions

In every group a leader will balance task and social–emotional functions and these in turn determine the range of roles to be adopted (see Figure 6.1). The **task functions** are activities carried out by a leader in order to enable a task to be achieved. Towards this goal the leader may act as: a) a teacher who is either didactic or simply a knowledgeable guide; b) someone who supplies equipment and resources; c) the person who plans the activity and structures the environment accordingly; d) someone who gives feedback to members on their performance. The **social–emotional functions** of a leader involve supporting members as needed. The leader will try to: a) give support and meet the needs of group members; b) enable communication and group interaction; c) encourage self expression in the group members; d) motivate the members; e) facilitate group spirit and cohesion.

The emphasis the leader gives to each function depends on the situation, namely, the type of group and the needs of members. In a craft group, for example, the leader will have to attend primarily to task functions, whereas the social aspects would be secondary. On the other hand, a psychotherapy

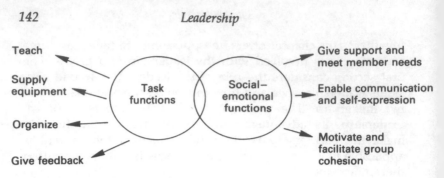

Figure 6.1 Group leader functions.

group will require the leader to focus mainly on the social–emotional functions. The leader in a drama therapy group will need to balance both functions when he or she teaches a particular technique and encourages members to participate.

Leader roles – activity groups

The leader of an activity group can play a multiplicity of roles encompassing both task and social–emotional functions. The roles adopted depend largely on the developmental level of the group and the needs of the members. Mosey's (1986) analysis of how to develop **group interaction skills**, described below, provides a structured approach to examining leader role behaviour.

In a **parallel group**, the therapist is very active as individuals at this level are unable to play many group membership roles. The therapist selects basic level activities, helps to carry them out, and in addition, meets members' needs for safety, love, acceptance and esteem. The leader will also reinforce desired behaviour in members such as engaging in the task, answering a question and recognizing another member. The leader will shape members' behaviour by giving praise and ignoring inappropriate behaviour.

The leader of a group operating at the **project level** helps members to begin to select activities which are short-term and require some interaction. The leader continues to take responsibility for planning the activity and meeting members' needs. At this level the therapist reinforces behaviour when two or more members work together or interact.

For the **ego-centric cooperative group**, the therapist takes on much less of a director role and acts more as a role model, trying to allow the group to function more independently. The therapist will reinforce any behaviours which are helpful for longer term tasks. Group members are more responsible for organizing their activities though the therapist may make suggestions and give assistance. The therapist helps members to meet each other's needs for recognition and esteem, whilst continuing to meet their love and safety needs.

The therapist in a **cooperative group** will usually act as either an advisor or participant. As an advisor, the therapist may initially set up the group and then withdraw, being available for consultation and support when necessary. As a participant, the therapist and group members have a mutual responsibility for the group activities and reinforcing behaviour.

The leader of a **mature group** acts as a group member as much as possible. The therapist will only take on those group membership roles which are necessary at a particular time. The leader will ensure the members give each other opportunity to experiment safely with roles.

Leader roles – support groups

Yalom (1975) identifies three fundamental tasks for a leader in a psychotherapy group: a) the creation and maintenance of the group; b) culture building; c) activation and process illumination. I would add a fourth task: d) handling transference. These four tasks give a good baseline to discuss the roles a leader adopts in any support group.

Creation and maintenance of the group

Yalom asserts that the leader is solely responsible for creating and convening the group. As the group starts, the leader assumes a gate-keeping function, encouraging members to stay or adding members as necessary. The therapist seeks to deter any forces which threaten the cohesion of the group such as scapegoating, sub-grouping or member absences. Finally, as members only know each other initially through the leader, he or she is the group's primary unifying force and assumes the role of 'transitional object'.

Culture building

The therapist then shapes the group into a therapeutic social system, guiding the formation of norms and group interaction. The therapist acts as both a technical expert (for instance employing facilitative techniques to encourage members to speak) and as a model participant, who sets norms by example (such as being non-judgemental or taking the risk to confront others). Yalom (1976, p 109) stresses that a leader is always communicating something which will impact on the group culture. As an example of this, he describes a therapist who ignores late-comers and so gives a non-welcoming message, thereby promoting a non-caring culture.

Activation and process illumination

The most complex role played by a psychotherapeutic group leader involves moving the group into the 'here-and-now' to highlight inter-group relationships and processes. The leader is centrally involved in offering a 'process commentary' to guide self-reflection. Here, the leader has to first recognize under-lying group dynamics and not simply respond directly to comments made. Second, the leader invites members to be aware of their own processes, and search for methods to facilitate self-knowledge rather than impose interpretations.

Dealing with transference

Transference is most closely identified with psychotherapy, though occurs in all therapy situations. It is an unconscious process where a person responds to another in a manner similar to the way he or she responded to a significant person in the past. In other words, feelings for another are **trans-ferred** – often onto the therapist. As Yalom (1976, p 191) summarizes, 'feelings transferred are "false connections", new editions of old impulses'. For instance, a group member may become dependent on a therapist, translating his or her need for a nurturing mother onto the therapist. Another member may respond to the group leader with hostility, perceiving the leader as an authority figure and transferring angry feelings normally felt towards his or her father. As Yalom (1976, p 195)

THEORY INTO PRACTICE

Process illumination

In a women's support group six members are involved as well as two leaders, one male and one female. At the beginning of the third session, after a brief, embarrassed silence, one member, Daisy, turns to the female leader and says 'Ask some questions to get us started'. If the leader was to simply respond to the spoken content, she could ask some facilitating questions, but in doing so, she might miss some critical underlying dynamic. The leader would be better placed if she considered the statement from several perspectives. Consider the possible dynamics which might underlie Daisy's simple request.

1. Could Daisy be expressing her own wish to ask questions of the group members? Would this be her way of disclosing aspects of herself?
2. How much is Daisy trying to control the rest of the group and how it is to proceed? By asking the therapist to control the events she de-powers the rest of the group. How do other members respond – do they allow this?
3. Is Daisy expressing her need to be dependent? Does this signal dependence on the therapist to initiate events?
4. Is the request a defensive plea to protect the group from its own processes? Is it an effort to avoid a tense silence?
5. How relevant is it that Daisy asks for the female leader's contribution rather than the male leader's ideas? With all the group members being female, the one male (who is also a leader) is bound to arouse feelings and be a focus for projections.
6. Why does Daisy ask one therapist rather than the other? Is this her way of punishing the other therapist who had challenged her the week before?
7. If Daisy is chiefly intent on attacking the male therapist, why does she proceed so indirectly? Is this her characteristic way of expressing anger?

---

explains, 'Every patient to a greater or lesser degree, perceives the therapist incorrectly because of transference distortions. Few are conflict-free in their attitudes toward such issues as parental authority, dependency, God, autonomy and rebellion

– all of which often come to be personified in the person of the therapist.'

Our therapist role in handling transference is threefold:

1. We need to recognize the possibility of transference processes occurring within any group. When we spot this happening, it can be a valuable source of information. If, for
instance, a group member is continually talking to the leader
and seeking a response, might he or she be seeking approval
from or wanting to be dependent on the therapist?

2. It helps to be aware of our own responses to clients and any
counter-transference in action. A therapist might find him or
her self for example, being uncharacteristically authoritarian.
This might be related to a client's own difficulty handling
authority. As another example, a female therapist may be feeling
'blocked' and 'put-down' by a male member. The therapist
might wonder if this reaction is something she commonly feels,
if so, this is a personal issue for the therapist to work on
outside the group.

3. If transference is identified, our next role as therapist is
to help members work through the process. Yalom (1976)
explains this can be achieved through: a) **consensual validation**
(testing the reality of a feeling, attitude or behaviour against
other member reactions); b) **therapist transparency**, where
the therapist reveals more of him or herself, which allows
members to confirm or change their impressions.

Leader responsibilities

As group leaders, we have certain responsibilities in relation to
the group and its members. Whittaker (1985) outlines the
responsibilities as being to, in and for any group. The leader's
responsibility **to** the group involves working to the best of his
or her ability for the benefit of group members. **Within** the
group, the leader has responsibility to be clear about its aims,
methods and processes and to behave accordingly. The leader
is not solely responsible **for** the group, but carries more
responsibility than the members (for example, the leader needs
to attend every group).

Benson (1987) suggests a leader has a responsibility to
communicate what he calls 'the three C's': a) **Competency** – the

leader should know what he or she is doing. This does not preclude feeling anxious or uncertain, it just means not being overwhelmed by these feelings. b) **Compassion** – the leader should demonstrate consideration, care and compassion, showing members he or she wants to understand and be involved. c) **Commitment** – the leader needs to believe in the efficacy of the group and its methods. Benson stresses the importance of the leader never imposing experiences onto a group which he or she is not prepared to experience as well.

The issue of power. I would extend Benson's analysis to suggest we have a responsibility not to abuse our power as a leader. When we lead a group, we are in a position to influence and control it. We set the agenda and so wield a considerable degree of power. It could be said that when we set out to 'facilitate', 'shape' or 'change' behaviour, we are exercising power by manipulating others. Power issues are complicated and can be difficult to handle, so it is important that we are clear about our attitudes and position concerning our power. Some points relevant to the extent and limits of our power are suggested below – do you agree with them?

Firstly, we usually have power over group members in the form of what Whittaker (1985) calls 'fate-control'. She notes we are in a position to influence decisions about members treatment and future (for instance we influence discharge dates). At a more immediate level, we can control who attends the group and who should be excluded.

Secondly, power is invested in us as leaders, by group members. As Whittaker (1985, p 375) describes, 'Persons in groups not infrequently assume that a leader has more or different powers than he actually has, and develop fantasies about the destructive or magically helpful ways. in which he might or could use his power.' These expectations are important as members behave accordingly. For instance, if members believe a leader will cure them, then they are likely to passively wait for the leader to act.

Thirdly, there are real limits to our power. We cannot force people to feel or behave in certain ways or to conform to our expectations of how the group ought to work. We cannot 'cure' our patients or force them to benefit from our group. In a different way, we may lack control as a group leader, when outside agents hold the power. Different examples of this are: the patient who is discharged without our agreement; the group member who is called away from the group to have another treatment; the parents who refuse to bring their child in for treatment.

LEADERSHIP STYLES

What is your leadership style? Can you adopt a different approach according to the situation? What style best suits different therapeutic situations? To explore these questions, this section will examine some key research on leadership styles and contrast directive versus non-directive styles used in groupwork.

THEORY INTO PRACTICE

Assessing leadership behaviour

Consider the following behaviours written in the form of bi-polar constructs. Place a tick along each continuum to identify the extent to which you demonstrate that behaviour as a leader of a particular group. If you display both characteristics equally, place your tick in the middle. You may find it useful to compare your ticks for different groups as you probably adapt your style to suit the situation. As a different exercise you could compare your style with that of another leader (perhaps your co-leader).

directive .... non-directive
creative .... practical
talkative .... quiet
confronting .... encouraging
contained .... enthusiastic
passive .... active
initiating .... cooperating
non-judgemental .... evaluative
self-disclosing .... reserved
task orientated .... socially orientated
ideas orientated .... details orientated
permissive .... controlling
group centred .... self centred

Some research on leadership

In their much quoted pioneering series of studies, Lewin, Lippitt and White (1939) investigated three alternative styles of leadership: authoritarian, democratic and laissez-faire. Lewin *et al.* arranged for three groups of boys and girls to make masks. One group was led by a leader who adopted an **authoritarian** style and issued orders; the second by a **democratic** leader who got the children to discuss what they wanted to do and how to achieve their objectives; the final group worked with a **laissez-faire** leader who was present but did not initiate any action.

The experiment demonstrated that the authoritarian group produced more work over a shorter period, but the children were resentful and dissatisfied. Some became aggressive, others retreated into apathy. Further, originality was inhibited and dependence stimulated. The democratically led group became more productive as they learned how to cooperate with each other and use the resources well. Motivation and satisfaction remained high and participants enjoyed the group. The laissez-faire group was neither productive or satisfied. They spent a disproportionate amount of time discussing their task which led to frustration and some aggression. Lewin *et al.* subsequently told the leaders to change their style which similarly affected the outcome. They also switched two of the more aggressive children who, in another group, became cooperative.

The main conclusions of this classic study are that leadership style will dramatically affect a group and that a leader can be trained to adopt a relevant style. The heavy bias towards democratic leadership of this result does, however, need to be understood in terms of the social context of the time which strongly favoured democracy above autocracy.

Fiedler (1968) offers a more interactionist perspective. He developed a model of leadership effectiveness which suggests that a leader's performance is contingent on the 'fit' between psychological and situational variables (see Figure 6.2). The **psychological variables** affecting performance include: a) style, such as being more directive and controlling or permissive and accepting; b) personal attributes, such as the ability to make judgements. The **situational variables** consider: a) the quality

Psychological	**Situational**
Style e.g. controlling or permissive	Relationships, e.g. liking between members
Attributes e.g. organizational ability	The type of task
	Power position and authority of leader

Figure 6.2 Variables influencing leader's performance.

THEORY INTO PRACTICE

Authoritarian, democratic, laissez-faire leaders – a group training exercise

The task: This is a fantasy role play which aims to stimulate wider discussion about leadership styles, and be fun. Divide the learners into three groups. Each will have a leader who adopts a different style. The role play scene involves being on a space ship which is going to blow up in 10 minutes and only one person can be saved. Members then argue for their survival.

Expected outcome: Whilst this exercise results in different group behaviours it is interesting to note certain regularities. Often the authoritarian group is quickest to come to a decision, though this changes if the crew revolt and overthrow the captain. The laissez-faire group either becomes apathetic or appoints a new leader. The democratic leader and method is usually accepted by the group.

Discussion points: 1) Who was saved and why? How was the decision made? 2) How did the group respond to the leader? Would this occur in real life? 3) What are the different ways (positive and negative) people respond to each type of leadership?

---

of leader and member relationships, which includes degree of mutual liking and respect; b) the task, such as its degree of structure and complexity; c) the power position of the leader, which includes the extent to which the leader can reward or punish members and the authority invested in the leader by the members.

Simply put, Fiedler's research reminds us that our leadership style both affects and is affected by the group. Further, the leader's behaviour cannot be separated from the wider social context or from people's perceptions of that situation. More specifically it suggests that leaders who are managing and controlling perform effectively in either very favourable or unfavourable situations, whilst considerate, permissive leaders operate best in semi-favourable conditions (for instance where the leader is liked but where there is a difficult task to do).

Lewin's and Fiedler's work present contrasting arguments. Firstly, Lewin considers leadership style can be adopted, whereas Fiedler sees style as involving stable personality characteristics. Secondly, unlike Lewin, Fiedler stresses the importance of the social context. Thirdly, Lewin maintains that leaders can be trained to lead, whilst Fiedler argues that leaders should be selected to fit a particular situation. Thus, theories of leadership are relevant as each perspective carries different practical implications.

Directive versus non-directive leadership

In therapy groups it is common to distinguish between directive and non-directive leadership styles. The **directive** style is most often adopted for activity groups where the leader instructs members on how to carry out a work or social activity. This style can be seen along an authoritarian–democratic continuum. At one end, the group leader controls and dictates each step of the group activity. At the other end, the leader guides and encourages members to participate in a certain direction.

The **non-directive** style is tied to a basic philosophy of human potential which stresses the capacity within each individual to be self-directed. The approach is most closely associated with counselling and psychotherapy groups, where members choose their own level of social and emotional participation. Non-directiveness can be plotted along the democratic-laissez-faire spectrum, where the leader will have differing degrees of control over, and responsibility for, the group. The laissez-faire leader tends to be non-directive and

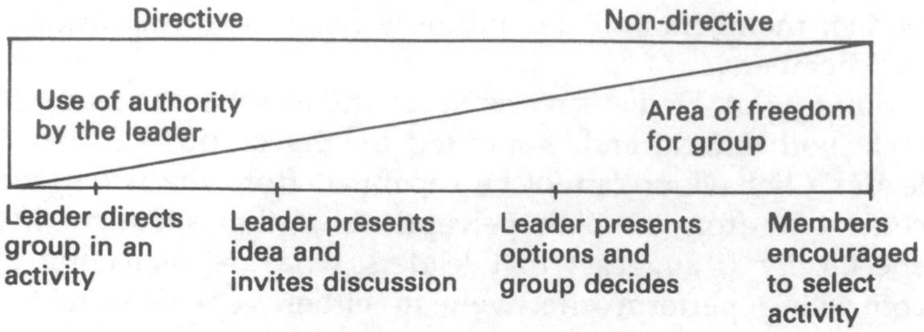

Figure 6.3 Leader styles and group responsibility (modified version of one presented by Howe and Swartzberg, 1986, p 113).

lets the group members set their own agenda. The democratic leader might set the scene but then let the group members make their own decisions about what and how much to share.

THEORY INTO PRACTICE

Collage group activity – directive and non-directive leader styles

A **directive** leader decides that the activity will be a group collage using cut-out magazine pictures of food. The leader sets out the relevant equipment, directs each member to tear out any pictures they see of food. The leader then allocates roles to members according to their skill levels, for instance, three members cut out the pictures, two paste, three others design the layout. The leader is active and encourages group involvement, sharing and interaction. Benefits of this approach are: i) successful end product ii) graded group interaction practice iii) members all involved in task.

A **non-directive** leader lays out a range of materials including lentils, magazines, paper, glue, plus some samples of past collages made. The leader asks what collage the group would like to make. The leader hands over responsibility to the group, is accepting of people's contributions and joins in as instructed by the members. Benefits of this approach are: i) creativity is stimulated ii) members are encouraged to take responsibility for themselves iii) self-esteem is raised as trust for decision making is handed over.

Directive group therapy

A more directive style is adopted when either the group needs to achieve an end product, or the members require limits to contain their behaviour. Often, the less able the members are to interact and make decisions, the more directive the leader needs to become. It cannot be emphasized enough, however, that directiveness is not synonymous with making decisions for the group members. Rather, being directive is structuring the group activity to encourage involvement and learning.

A particularly good illustration of directive group therapy comes from Kathy Kaplan (1988) where she advocates a specific treatment called 'Directive Group' to meet the needs of acutely ill, minimally functioning psychiatric patients. Suitable patients show marked difficulties in simple task performance, self care and basic interaction. They exhibit extremes of behaviours, for example, are passive, aggressive, withdrawn or confused.

For Kaplan, the term directive refers to the active way a leader structures the environment and activity to ensure maximum member participation.

The Directive Group can be summarized with reference to four components: a) **structure** – six to ten patients attend with two co-leaders who '. . . provide role models for action, support and collaborative interaction.' (Kaplan, 1988, p 25). The group meets daily at a routine time and place for 45 minutes. Most patients attend for at least a week. A predictable sequence of events (orientation, introduction, warm-up activities, selected activities, wrap up) helps minimize patient problems of confusion. b) **Theoretical framework** – the group is based on the model of human occupation which helps to conceptualize patients' functioning level. c) **Goals** – group and individual goals are presented. Four group goals encourage cohesion by emphasizing participation and interaction. Ten more are compatible individual patient goals (such as 'make one comment on own per group'). d) **Activities** – the group's activities include the wide range of games, crafts, movement and communication exercises adapted for the basic skill level of the patients.

Non-directive group therapy

A more non-directive style is adopted when group members are able to use their own resources, and in effect, take on their own leadership roles. The leader is responsible for monitoring and using what is happening in the group and follows the group's lead. The leader responds to the group at their level of understanding and avoids interpretation. This allows members to come to their own conclusions and understanding. Note that the non-directive leader is active, rather than passive, indeed the non-directive group might be better termed 'self-directed'.

The most influential authority on the non-directive approach is Carl Rogers (1970). He developed the non-directive counselling technique, the philosophy of which he applied to encounter and psychotherapy groups. His approach has been widely applied in the range of humanistic therapies. Virginia Axline (1989) is one disciple who became an authority on applying the principles to **play therapy** with children. She advocates group play therapy for children whose problems are centred on social adjustment. 'The group experience injects into therapy a very realistic element because the child lives in the world with other children and must consider the reaction of others and must develop a consideration of other individuals' feelings' (Axline, 1989, p 23).

Axline lays down eight basic principles to guide a non-directive therapist:

1. The therapist must develop a warm, friendly relationship with the child, in which good rapport is established as soon as possible.
2. The therapist accepts the child exactly as he or she is.
3. The therapist establishes a feeling of permissiveness in the relationship so that the child feels free to express his or her feelings completely.
4. The therapist is alert to recognize the feelings the child is expressing and reflects those back in such a manner that the child gains insight into his or her behaviour.
5. The therapist maintains a deep respect for the child's ability to solve his or her own problems if given the opportunity to do so. The responsibility to make choices and to institute change is the child's.
6. The therapist does not attempt to direct the child's actions

THEORY INTO PRACTICE

Identify your own group leading style*

If you were leading the following groups, which approach(es) would you most likely adopt? If none of the approaches suit you, select d) and note what would be your chosen response.

1. In a craft group, one patient continually talks which prevents others from contributing their ideas. Would you:
   a) ask the patient to talk less to allow others to participate more?
   b) try to re-direct the conversation and encourage others to speak?
   c) wait for other group members to handle the situation?
   d) do none of the above?

2. In a business meeting, a few members are getting side-tracked onto irrelevant issues and distracted from the task at hand. Would you:
   a) join in the irrelevant discussion as the team seems to need this to occur and you do not wish to take control at this point?
   b) encourage members to focus on the agenda items?
   c) ask the distractors to keep to the point?
   d) do none of the above?

3. In a drama therapy group, one client remains silent and does not share her experiences unless directly prompted. Would you:
   a) say and do nothing. You accept her silence as her right not to commit herself to the group at this stage?
   b) say you would like to hear from her?
   c) employ group exercises which encourage verbal participation?
   d) do none of the above?

4. In a staff planning meeting, one member seems hostile to you as leader and continually disagrees with your suggestions without offering alternatives. Would you:
   a) ask the member to stop only disagreeing with you and offer some constructive suggestions instead?
   b) ignore it initially and wait to see how the other members react. If it continues, express your own feelings in return?

   c) summarize the point of disagreement and ask what
      other members feel?

   d) do none of the above?

5. One of your staff members comes in persistently late for
   the weekly meeting. As the head of department, if you
   were to handle this situation in the group, would you:
   a) ask the staff member to try to be on time next week?
   b) state your view in general that it is important members
      are punctual for meetings?
   c) ignore it and hope peer pressure will take effect?
   d) do none of the above?

6. In a group discussion, a fairly prolonged argument develops between two members. Would you:
   a) summarize the two viewpoints and open up the dis-
      cussion to other members?
   b) only intervene if the situation gets out of control as you
      believe members should be allowed to express nega-
      tive aspects?
   c) ask the members to stop arguing as it is no longer
      constructive?
   d) do none of the above?

7. In the first of a series of supportive psychotherapy sessions, as facilitator would you start the group by saying:
   a) This is our group, we can make the experience into
      what we wish?
   b) Let us start by each of us introducing ourselves and
      saying one thing we hope to gain from the group?
   c) The aims of the group are for us to explore feelings and
      to gain awareness of ourselves and others?
   d) do none of the above?

The three approaches given for each situation loosely high-
lights a particular style of leadership, namely directive, democratic and non-directive. Compare your answers to the key
below.

1. a) directive	b) democratic	c) non-directive
2. a) non-directive	b) democratic	c) directive
3. a) non-directive	b) directive	c) democratic
4. a) directive	b) non-directive	c) democratic
5. a) directive	b) democratic	c) non-directive
6. a) democratic	b) non-directive	c) directive
7. a) non-directive	b) directive	c) democratic

Discussion: Does any one style predominate your responses? Do you move between styles depending on the situation? If you selected d) on any items, what does your response reveal about your style?

* Questionnaire based on a similar idea as one printed in Priestley and McGuire (1983, pp 136–138)

or conversation in any manner. The child leads the way; the therapist follows.

7. The therapist does not attempt to hurry the therapy along. It is a gradual process and is recognized as such by the therapist.

8. The therapist establishes only those limitations that are necessary to anchor the therapy to the world of reality and to make the child aware of his or her responsibility in the relationship. (Axline, 1989, pp 69–70).

CO-LEADERSHIP

Co-leadership involves complex processes which extend beyond simply duplicating one leader's role. For a start, different patterns of co-leadership can occur, such as having two leaders or a leader and a support co-leader who takes less responsibility. Some groups benefit from multiple leadership and other groups do not. The partners need to be able to work together, support each other and negotiate their differences. Their relationship then has an impact on the group and subsequent dynamics. This section will explore some of these complexities, examining in turn: the criteria for deciding to co-lead; its advantages and disadvantages; considerations for selecting a co-worker; and how to make the co-leader relationship work.

The decision to co-lead

Are groups more effective with two leaders? Do certain types of groups do better with one leader? Can it be useful to have several leaders? To lead or co-lead a group? . . . these are the questions and there are no clear-cut answers. Little research has been carried out on the relative effectiveness of leading groups alone or with co-therapists. Groupworkers seem to differ in their opinions about which is best. However, co-leadership should not occur simply as a matter of tradition or because of an unwillingness to work alone. Ideally, the decision of whether or not to work with a co-leader should be a positive one, based on a judgement about group needs and the effectiveness of the partnership.

Group needs

Activity groups are fairly flexible and can tolerate sole or multiple leadership. One leader may be all that is required for a basic activity group consisting of three to nine patients or clients, but two or more leaders (or support staff) would be advantageous if one-to-one teaching or attention is required by group members. In larger activity groups, where work may take place in sub-groups, several leaders can be helpful providing members do not feel de-powered (for example, picking up the message they are unable to monitor their own sub-group) or intimidated (by feeling constantly observed). As a general rule fewer staff leaders are needed where the patients and clients can take on leadership roles themselves.

In **support groups**, where the emphasis is on socio-emotional aspects, it is best to have two leaders. Having two leaders, or at least one leader and another person who acts as 'support staff', offers a safety net for the group, in that one leader can hold the group together whilst the other is freed to work with individuals as needed. Two or more leaders allows for better evaluation of the group as one leader can be freed to monitor overall processes if another is caught up with emotions of the moment. However, care must be taken to keep staff numbers down. Two co-leaders and a student observer, for instance, might be acceptable in a group of eight clients but would over-power four.

Effectiveness of the partnership

The success or failure of a group can be determined by how well the co-leaders inter-relate and combine as a partnership –

THEORY INTO PRACTICE

Sole or multiple leadership? Different needs for different groups

Consider the different examples of groups below. Note the different patterns of leadership adopted. Do you agree with the decision made about leadership and the rationale offered? What other information do you need in order to come to a clear decision about the most effective leadership pattern for that group?

Group leadership arrangement	Rationale
1. Social skills training group: – 6 clients and 3 staff involved. – Two therapists act as co-leaders. – They take equal responsibility to plan and run the group. – One student takes a listening role in the planning sessions and acts as a 'stooge' in the role plays.	i) The two leaders work well together as their styles complement each other (one is forceful and the other is gently supportive). ii) The stooge role is useful enabling leaders to be observers in the role plays. iii) Student needs to observe a group in action but does not have the experience to lead.
2. Baking group: – 5 clients and 1 staff member – staff member works alongside group members and encourages them to take responsibility.	i) One staff member only is necessary for safety reasons. ii) Group members can assume their own leader roles.
3. Reality orientation group: – 5 patients and 4 staff members – Each staff member takes turns to lead the group whilst the others work alongside individual patients. – All staff are involved with planning the group.	i) The patients tend to wander and need one-to-one attention. ii) Having several staff involved enables them to give each other support. This is a tiring, demanding group.

it is perhaps more important than establishing the acceptable number of leaders. Generally, four conditions need to be met for a partnership to work: i) one leader's skills and personality should not simply duplicate that of the other; ii) beliefs, values or theoretical stances of the leaders should be complementary; iii) the leaders need to like and feel comfortable with each other in a working relationship; iv) the leaders must respect each other's contributions. If these conditions cannot be met it is better for leaders to work alone.

Advantages and disadvantages of co-leadership

Co-leadership offers three main ADVANTAGES which are of benefit to both group and leaders involved. First, co-leadership can increase the **effectiveness of a group**. Some groups are easier to manage with two leaders, particularly where members need close supervision or containment, or when difficult behaviours such as withdrawal or acting out are involved. One therapist can work with the individuals as needed, whilst the other manages the group as a whole. At a more subtle level, the effectiveness of the groupwork may be increased by two therapists if they offer complementary approaches. One therapist may be more supportive to members, whilst the other takes on a challenging role. Alternatively, when one therapist is stuck or blocked by transference processes, the other leader can become more active and counterbalance any effects.

Second, co-working can provide much needed **mutual support** and encouragement to the leaders, particularly when one of the partnership is lacking confidence or is confused about the group dynamics and how to proceed. Pre-and post-group discussions offer the opportunity for leaders to explore (and off-load) their feelings and gain comfort from someone else who also experienced the group. For difficult groups, the support of another's presence can help decrease anxiety and give an added protection at both a practical and emotional level.

Third, co-leadership is a direct and valuable opportunity **to develop each other's professional skills** and a greater understanding of groups. Therapists can model on and learn from each other. The post-group discussions between leaders will often clarify what occurred in the group. A partner can also increase therapist objectivity, which is particularly important in psychotherapy, where a therapist is often trying to untangle what is real as opposed to counter-transference distortion.

Each of these benefits are important in their own right. When a partnership works well and the leaders are in tune, the advantages of co-leadership are amplified. If, however, the leaders are ill-matched or unprepared, the disadvantages are quickly revealed.

The main DISADVANTAGES of running a group with two or more leaders are the increased **demands of time and resources**. Two therapists are twice as expensive as one, and more to the point, preparation time is disproportionately increased. The co-leaders not only need to be able to take the time to run the group, but they need additional opportunities to negotiate when planning and to give each other feedback and support.

A poor or unplanned co-leadership combination can **create problems for the group**. The leaders may be at cross purposes with each other regarding goals or approach, which is not only confusing for membership but could well undermine therapeutic aims. One example of this occurred in an evaluation group. The more experienced therapist was concerned to encourage the clients to evaluate their own improvements. The less experienced co-leader inadvertently undermined this process by giving her own view on the members gains first.

A third source of problem arises where there is a clash of **conflicting leadership styles**. This was evident in one discussion group where one leader was inclined to be talkative which directly opposed the others' view that therapists should be relatively passive in the group. Tensions escalated as the therapists did not give each other feedback. The quieter therapist became increasingly irritated and started to intervene in the discussions before his partner could. The unfortunate result was a group over-dominated by both leaders.

A fourth kind of problem arises when the leaders deploy **contradictory theoretical orientations**. Consider the likely confusions which would result for members if one therapist attempts to establish an accepting, encouraging environment, whilst the other is more critical and concerned with achieving end-products. All these negative group experiences could be avoided with only one leader or if the leaders took time to negotiate their role and interventions.

Selecting a co-leader

The potential advantages and disadvantages of co-leadership flags up the importance of selecting a compatible co-leader. So, what qualities are needed for an effective partnership? The research literature suggests that leaders should examine their values, professional status and gender mix.

Values

It is essential for co-leaders to **believe in** the group and what they are doing as a partnership. The leaders need to share similar views about their aims, expectations and approach to the group and its members. What would be the likely outcome, for instance, of a social skills training group where one of the leaders dislikes role play and would prefer to be involved in a psychotherapy group? If the group members pick up on this lack of commitment their own involvement would diminish. The leaders would need to carefully examine their attitudes prior to the group beginning. The leaders may then decide that a social skills group is inappropriate, or they may find a compromise, such as, the reluctant leader shares with the group his or her difficulties about role play whilst still participating.

Whilst it is not necessary for the co-leaders to share exactly the same **theoretical orientation**, their views still need to be complementary. To illustrate this, think about the impact on a self-awareness art group where one group leader is inclined towards analytical ways of working, whilst the other is humanistic. A **negative scenario** could arise in which the analytical therapist attempts to interpret the members paintings in conflict with the other who is aiming to encourage free expression. The result is that the group members are confused about what is expected of them. Perhaps worst of all, the therapists do not take the time to re-evaluate their aims and approach. In contrast to this, a **positive scenario** might envisage both therapists agreeing to ask the group members for their understanding of their own paintings. The analytical therapist would not directly interpret the paintings but might offer some tentative ideas. The leaders could then use their post-group discussion to air their different interpretations.

Professional status

The status of the leaders (including their position, background and experience) needs to be taken into account as inequalities in the relationship can create problems. This is particularly relevant to occupational therapy groups as the experience level of leaders often varies, for instance, therapists regularly work with students and support staff.

Research into co-leader mix recommends that leaders should be of **equal** status and experience in order to benefit from mutual feedback and stimulation, and for group members to experience their combined skill. Otherwise co-leaders can be unsettled by an unequal relationship. One leader may feel unduly pressured to continually perform and take more of the lead whilst the other feels increasingly inadequate with less to offer – and so it escalates. If the relationship is an unequal one, the leaders need to work out a clear division of labour where each feels comfortable and has a positive role to play. The senior partner can teach by modelling and encouragement, and the learner avoid either being overly competitive or non-assertive.

Differences in professional backgrounds between leaders (say therapist and instructor) need not be a problem. However, difficulties can arise when group members **perceive** an inequality. The person who is perceived as less able or less respected is likely to feel de-skilled and defensive. Leaders should consider this possibility and take some pre-emptive action. One good example of this was the occasion when I (as a female occupational therapist) co-led a group with a (male) psychiatrist. We predicted the members would over-invest in the doctor. To counterbalance this undesirable effect, we decided that I should introduce and conclude each group in order to reinforce a stronger leader position for myself.

THEORY INTO PRACTICE

Negotiating roles – examples of alternative divisions of labour

TWO THERAPISTS – a life skills group: Both leaders aim to play an equal and active part. They will take turns introducing and running an activity. When one takes the lead, the other acts as a stooge in a role play or works with individuals as necessary.

A THERAPIST AND A TECHNICIAN – a pottery group: The technician is given responsibility for teaching the pottery techniques and organizing the work. The therapist facilitates group interaction. Having discussed the possibilities with the technician, the therapist plans the group activity and structures the environment to meet the treatment aims.

A THERAPIST AND A STUDENT – a creative therapy group: The therapist plans to take on the leader role. The student will act primarily as a member of the group, who in addition, will act as a model for the members. Although the therapist assumes the main responsibility for planning the group, the student gives suggestions and is active in the post-group discussions. The student also writes up the notes on the group with the therapist acting as supervisor.

Gender

Whilst research suggests that the gender mix of co-leaders is an important variable, it seems less relevant for many occupational therapy groups. As our profession is predominantly female, many of our groups automatically involve female leaders. If a choice is available, the decision about gender mix should be made on both practical and emotional grounds.

At the **practical level**, some groups may require a male–female combination, for instance, when faced with personal care activities such as changing clothes at the swimming baths. Alternatively, some groups may respond best to a single gender partnership, such as an all women's group. There are no hard and fast rules and each group needs to be considered in its own right. At an **emotional level**, a male–female co-therapist team can have some unique advantages. Male–female combinations have most impact in psychotherapy groups as they can powerfully evoke a family image which in turn, allows fantasies about parents to be worked through. Yalom (1975, p 423) adds to this idea when he recognizes, '... patients may benefit from the model setting of a male–female pair working together collaboratively with mutual respect without the destructive competition, mutual derogation, exploitation or pervasive sexuality too often associated with male–female pairings by the patient.'

Apart from these specific examples, I would suggest that the gender mix need not carry any more weight than other social variables, namely, the leader's age, ethnicity or class. The best leader combination is one which allows different group members to relate to one or other therapist at some level.

In all, the most effective leadership combinations for occupational therapy groups are those where there is a complementary attitude between co-leaders, where they respect and feel comfortable with each other. This in turn will impact on the group. Co-leaders should not simply duplicate each others' characteristics, however. Some contrasts between leaders are beneficial. Therapists' differences (in status, gender or other attributes) allow them to learn from each other and supplement each others' contributions, whilst the members have a wider choice of leaders to whom they can relate. Whittaker (1985, p 96) summarizes this nicely when she emphasizes that 'co-leadership works best when the two leaders are clearly different persons, with different strengths and sensitivities, but where they share certain basic stances and values concerning the group.'

Making co-leadership work

Leaders need to spend time together to get to know and feel comfortable with each other before deciding to co-lead a group. Having agreed to co-lead, the group should be jointly planned and the co-leadership roles clearly established. This ensures that both leaders are committed to similar aims and are clear about the methods to be employed. It also means the group can continue as planned if one leader is absent.

Setting up the co-leader relationship is only the first step. The leaders will only work together effectively if they can communicate regularly and openly. They need to be able to

THEORY INTO PRACTICE

The 'split the leaders' game

<u>Background situation:</u> one male and one female therapist co-lead a supportive psychotherapy group which consists of all women. During one group, the women express their anger towards men in general. At the end of the group, the male therapist makes a slightly confronting remark which is interpreted by all the members and the female co-therapist, as being critical. In the following group, it appears that anger is being indirectly expressed to the male therapist.

<u>Two alternative scenarios:</u>

Split leaders – at the end of the first group, the female co-therapist does not express her feelings to her co-leader. She feels angry with him on the members' behalf. She also feels the group is being threatened as her co-leader's critical approach seems to be inhibiting the members, making them reluctant to speak. In the following group, when the members start to attack the male leader indirectly, she inadvertently joins in. The female leader invites the members to express their anger directly and give some honest feedback to the man. After this group, both therapists avoid talking about what occurred and why.

United leaders – the female leader gives her partner some feedback in their post-group discussion. They discuss the pros and cons of his intervention. The female therapist begins to value it more and can see that it provoked a response which could be usefully worked through. She wonders, however, about its timing, a criticism which the male therapist accepts. They decide that in the following group, if the members try to avoid the issue, they will raise it themselves. In the following group, when the members begin their indirect attack, the female therapist points out what they seem to be doing and why. After the group, the therapists explore how well they handled the situation. The female therapist is concerned that she may have inadvertently encouraged too much 'flack' for her co-leader. Also, she gives him support as it was clearly a difficult group for him.

share their ideas and feelings, and give each other feedback and support. Further, they will need to be able to examine any problems which arise, for instance, honestly exploring how members are being allowed to undermine or split the leader relationship.

Joint supervision sessions can be a useful, more formal method of developing the partnership. Supervision is particularly vital for psychotherapy groups as the leaders may need help to disentangle the complexities of group dynamics and transferences. For activity groups, a supervisor may be able to offer new perspectives on the group or activity ideas.

This chapter has explored the process of group leadership from a number of angles. It first examined the different roles and functions a leader has in occupational therapy groups, and in particular task versus social–emotional roles were noted. Then it considered directive, non-directive and democratic leadership styles and how these both affect and are affected by the group situation. The final section focused on co-leadership, when it is effective, how to avoid the problems that can arise and how continued communication is essential if the relationship is to work.

7

Managing problems within a group

All group leaders experience problems in their groups from time to time. These problems can occur either at an individual or at a group level. Sometimes individuals create difficulties for the group, for instance when a member is over-dominating. At other times, several group members or even the whole group can be the problem, as is the case when a group erupts in conflict.

When faced with a problem, ask yourself three questions – the answers may be revealing.

- **When is it a problem?** A group in conflict, for example, may involve honest, constructive debate and be a positive situation.
- **To whom is it a problem?** A silent group, for instance, may only be a problem to the leader who wishes for a different response, the other members may feel quite comfortable.
- **Why is the problem occurring?** The cause of a problem is often hard to disentangle as several interlinking factors may be involved. The activity, environment or leader's approach may be inappropriate. Alternatively, the source of the problem may lie within the group and in individual members who feel destructive or negative.

This chapter explores seven common problems which confront us in groups. Four difficult behaviours that occur in individuals are discussed, namely, the silent, over-dominating, distressed or angry, and unpredictable or bizarre member. The three group problems explored are the silent group, the apathetic group and the group in conflict.

Each of these problems is examined in terms of the nature of the problem and why it may be occurring, and then some problem-solving ideas are considered. There are no 'instant recipe' answers for any of the problems and different strategies may work at different times.

No discussion of problems can capture the rich dynamics which would be played out in any single group. So, as you read through each problem section, have a specific group in mind and ask yourself the three questions above: **When**, **To whom**, and **Why**, is it a problem? The problem solving solution you choose will then be appropriate to the needs of your particular group.

THE SILENT MEMBER

All group therapists have experienced the potentially difficult situation of having a silent member in the group. This person poses several problems. For one thing, he or she may go unnoticed and unhelped. Further, non-participation can escalate as a group norm which will increasingly drain the more talkative members. It can also be difficult for participating members who may resent the member for 'withholding' when they are disclosing personal details.

We must expect that some people will remain quiet in any one group. A problem for the group as such only arises if, over a longer period of time, members react negatively to that individual's lack of participation. Often, silent members will claim they are still involved in the group, actively listening to and gaining from others, but they do not feel they have anything to contribute at that point. This is an important line to assess – is the silence understandable and temporary or does it signal a problem?

There are a number of reasons why a person might remain silent in a group. He or she may be naturally shy and assume the 'quiet one' role within a group – a habit that is hard to break out of. Alternatively, the person may be feeling flat or depressed, lacking the drive or group skills to contribute. The silent member may feel anxious or threatened in the group and avoid participation, fearing the group's reaction if they did in fact join in. Sometimes the silence may signal non-participation and an active communication of resistance to being in the group. Finally, the silent member syndrome may in fact be created by other group members, for example, when dominant members do not allow the person space to speak.

Problem-solving ideas

The best technique to help a silent member is the one that tackles the underlying reasons for being silent. Any of the following ideas could prove effective.

1. **Accept** the silent member's behaviour and avoid pushing him or her to participate. Pushing a person can result in a game of defensive silence and works against building up a feeling of group trust. Assume the member will contribute when he or she feels ready to and safe enough, and in the meantime be quietly supportive.
2. See the person on an **individual basis** to check out his or her perspective of the situation and explore the behaviour. Is this his or her normal reaction in groups? Does he or she want to participate more? Is there any way that the leader can encourage more contributions?
3. Silent members should be encouraged to communicate **non-verbally** – nodding, for example, to demonstrate involvement. This is the first step to communicating group involvement to the other members. As the next step, a practical tip for people in the quiet role habit is to break it slowly by joining in with contributions like, 'I agree'.
4. It may be useful to tackle the problem more directly within the **group situation**, for instance saying, 'You've not expressed your view – what do you think?'. Or we might ask more generally, 'Those of you who haven't spoken yet, have you any other ideas to add?'
5. Regular use of pair and **smaller groupwork** can be a helpful technique to encourage member participation. Where appropriate, group members can be assigned particular roles which may specifically encourage silent members to take an active part. These roles can be real ones established for the maintenance of the group such as 'tea maker'. Alternatively, they may be artificially created, such as in role play, where the silent member is put into a more assertive or talkative role. Some exercises such as 'the gold fish bowl' (see Figure 7.1) could come into this category and often produce interesting results.
6. Group leaders should watch and consider their own be-

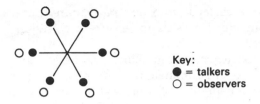

Key:
● = talkers
○ = observers

Figure 7.1 The goldfish bowl discussion.

haviour, especially **eye contact**. Well timed eye contact with quieter members may help them to speak. At a more subtle level, as leaders, we may be unconsciously reinforcing the silent member pattern by only encouraging the more talkative members.

THEORY INTO PRACTICE

The goldfish bowl discussion technique

The group members are divided into an inner circle and outer circle. The inner circle are involved in a group discussion whilst the outer circle observe and are not allowed to speak.

The choice of which members go into which circle is particularly relevant. The groups may be divided into men and women for example, to explore gender issues. Alternatively, quieter members may take the inner circle position and discuss their feelings about their level of participation. The inner circle provides a safer, more intimate forum which may encourage their participation. The more dominant members are forced to listen which also may help to even out levels of interaction.

THE DOMINATING MEMBER

In contrast to the previous problem behaviour, group leaders are frequently faced with the difficulty of having one or more over-dominating members in our group. Yalom (1975, p 376) calls the 'habitual monopolist' the 'bete noire' of many group therapists. By its nature this problem is often felt sooner and more acutely as other group members become quickly irritated and may well lapse into non-participation and apathy rather than compete. If this happens group cohesion can be quickly destroyed.

Occasionally, the group allows, and even encourages, one or two members to dominate the group as this gives space for the other members to opt out. Whittaker (1985) explains this process as a 'restrictive solution' whereby some members do not need to talk and expose themselves to risk if they can get another person to do this. Often this dynamic occurs in the early stages of a group, and as the group becomes more established the need for one person to dominate lessens.

The dominating member is often keen to participate but is so self-absorbed that he or she is unaware of others' needs. He or she is likely to jump in and respond first when a remark is made to the group and may take the opportunity to offer a long-winded personal story. More problematic is the member who talks constantly, even aggressively, and moralizes, offers advice and interrupts others. At the extreme, in a psychiatric setting a member in the throes of a manic or psychotic episode may be unable to control a stream of bizarre delusional talk.

The problem of a dominating member usually arises from a combination of factors. First, the member may be self-centred or simply may not appreciate the group rules of 'not hogging' the available space. Second, wider group dynamics may be involved with members actively encouraging the dominant behaviour. Third, in a linked way, the leader may have unduly encouraged the dominant member early on, feeling relieved someone was prepared to speak.

In any event, the leader needs to handle the situation sensitively and well. Other group members will be watching and waiting for something to be done. Even greater problems may arise if the leader is seen to reject the talker. This lessens trust and leaves other members feeling insecure that they may be 'put down' at a later date. Alternatively, if the leader is unable to control the behaviour he or she may be perceived as ineffective, again reducing trust.

Problem-solving ideas

1. Do not simply silence the person. **Examine** the behaviour, otherwise the person will not be able to learn new ways for

the future. It is also important to allow the talker his or her fair share of space.

2. It may be necessary to speak to the person on a **one-to-one** basis. Stress that you value his or her contributions but that it is also important to listen and learn from others. The person may well benefit from feedback about how he or she is being over-dominating and needs to increase awareness of other group members' needs.

3. As a group leader, you might try **sitting next to** the over-dominant member. This reduces eye contact and so does less to encourage participation. It also allows you to use short physical or verbal prompts such as a light restraining hand on the person's arm saying 'hang on, let's hear someone else'.

4. Sometimes, it may be possible to **draw other members** in by asking, for example, 'who agrees/disagrees?' with the points made by the over-participatory speaker. Equally, this can be turned round by asking the talker what other members' opinions might be. This provides an opportunity to suggest the need to make space to hear the other members' views.

5. Yalom (1975, p 379) commends a slightly paradoxical strategy of **encouraging** the member to say more! Compulsive speech in this context is seen as a defence, holding the group at arm's length and 'sacrificing the opportunity for therapy to his insatiable need for attention and control'. A modification of this paradoxical strategy is to encourage the over-talkative member 'to help' the other members speak more.

6. Finally, the other group members can be confronted with their responsibility. In other words, make it a **group problem** rather than scapegoating an individual. It can be powerful to ask the group 'Why do you keep letting 'X' speak so much?' Point out that the behaviour cannot exist without the group permitting one member to carry the burden of talk. Interventions like these will often startle more passive members into participation.

THE ANGRY OR DISTRESSED MEMBER

In most therapy contexts we are frequently confronted with an angry or distressed member – a member in pain who suddenly breaks down in tears or is aggressive. Whilst it may be a problem for the individual who is suffering, it can also be one for the group members (including the leader) who are likely to feel concerned, frightened and possibly distressed themselves as their own emotions are triggered.

When strong emotions are being expressed such as sadness or anger, we need to recognize what may be occurring and why. First, the individual may simply be expressing their distress or tension. This can be viewed positively in that the person feels safe enough to share difficult feelings. Of greater concern are the more extreme situations where the expressed emotions appear to be escalating out of control. The person who explodes suddenly may be too mentally unstable to operate within an occupational therapy group.

Second, we should consider if the person is simply reacting to having emotions provoked by the treatment activity itself or reacting to other group members. Every therapy situation is a potentially powerful one which can be fraught with emotions. As therapists we need to feel confident that we can handle emotions that are expressed if we set out to facilitate their expression. It is professionally irresponsible, for instance, to run a projective art group asking members to explore deep feelings and then feel unable to deal with the group members and emotional material when it comes out. We should be wary of, whilst not avoid, using activities and techniques which can provoke strong feelings.

Third, a member may be expressing emotions on behalf of the group, having picked up the underlying group feeling. An example of this occurs when a rather tense group is not expressing feelings so one person 'rescues' the situation by suddenly crying. This person may well be expressing, unconsciously, a group need.

Problem-solving ideas

Whilst every emotional situation must be handled according to the needs of the individuals concerned, there are some rules of thumb which can be applied to most situations.

1. Initially it is important simply to **listen** to the distress being expressed – understand before intervening. In this way

we give permission, space and time for people to express feelings. Note how easy it can be, for instance, to stop someone crying by immediately cuddling them. However, this can also work the other way, when your show of sympathy results in an increase in the flow of tears!

2. As group leaders we need to manage our **own feelings**. We need to stay calm and not panic as most people experiencing distress are afraid of losing control. We need to be seen as being in control, able to protect the person and contain the feelings if necessary. We must also watch for any feelings of guilt for having provoked the emotions, as this may interfere with our judgement.

3. We have to consider the **specific needs** of the member concerned. If, for example, he or she is crying, it is best to leave a small respectful silence before asking if he or she wants to say anything more. If the person says no, he or she may well feel embarrassed about the public outburst so it is important to move on. If discussion is necessary, it can be postponed for a while and then returned to when the person feels more composed. This is invariably a safer way of handling the situation and can be more productive.

4. The line we seek is to encourage **constructive** rather than destructive expressions of emotion. For instance, if an angry outburst involves attacking another member, it needs to be controlled and handled. Another destructive situation which needs to be managed occurs when an individual leaves the group in high distress and is in danger of harming him or herself.

5. When a group member rushes out of the room in distress, group leaders are confronted with a dilemma. Should we as the leader stay with the group or rush out to help support the individual? If we are working with a co-therapist this is less of a problem as he or she can leave to speak with the upset member. The crunch comes when we are leading the group alone. In fact, there is only one answer to this dilemma – **our responsibility** is for the group so we must stay.* As a compromise, we might suggest another group

---

* Note if a patient is on a Section and requires constant supervision, we have to follow him or her. For this reason I would not have this individual in the group unless he or she was accompanied by another therapist or nurse.

member goes out and tries to give support. Having been in this problematic situation a number of times I have become more philosophical. If someone rushes out he or she may need this 'flight' to gain some space and is likely to return to the group when ready.

6. It may be necessary to see the distressed member on an **individual basis** or refer him or her on to another therapist. However, this can prove to be a problematic decision. Consider the situation of a member involved in a psycho-therapy group who gets upset but is unable to explore it. What message does the group therapist give out if he or she recommends one-to-one therapy? The unintentional message received by the group members is that the group cannot be trusted and that individual therapy is more effective. Then the therapist is likely to be faced by an escalation of members each saying they cannot speak of their difficulties in the group. If a person must have indivi-dual treatment it should be arranged with another therapist, and if possible should not take place alongside the group treatment. Only occasionally might an individual require some extra focused work which is not relevant to the group situation, for instance, discussing an experience of being sexually abused within an activity session.

7. Finally, we need to attend to the **other group members** and encourage them to express their feelings either during or after the emotional outburst. The members may have felt frightened and need reassurance. Equally, they may be upset in their own right, having had emotions stirred up and so require time to ventilate their feelings.

MANAGING DISRUPTIVE OR BIZARRE BEHAVIOUR

Therapists leading groups within psychiatric settings are likely to encounter individuals who are disruptive and difficult to control. These individuals may be acutely ill and be experi-encing a psychotic illness which results in bizarre and unpre-dictable behaviour. One instance of this would be the person who accuses, irrationally, an innocent member of malicious intent. Alternatively, the individual may simply be preoccupied with his or her own needs and unconcerned about any effects of his or her odd behaviour on others.

Behaviours which come under the heading of disruptive or bizarre poses problems for the therapist as: i) the individual may be demanding so much attention that other members lose out; ii) the behaviour disrupts the flow of the group process; iii) the out-of-control situation may well distress and frighten other group members.

Problem-solving ideas

1. Consider carefully, whether or not the person is suitable for the group. The member may be so out of touch with reality, lacking in concentration and unaware of others' needs as to be unable to operate in a group setting. If the person's behaviour is unduly disruptive to the group process then he or she should be **excluded** and perhaps re-join at a later stage.
2. **Manage** the behaviour. For instance if the person is psychotic and their delusional material is breaking out, try to contain it and focus on what appears to be the real content of any feelings that are being expressed. Responding to a tirade about evil forces in the radiator, for example, a therapist may say 'I can't see these forces but I can see you feel frightened of them.'
3. Attend to the **degree of stimulation** and pressure within the environment and group activity. A concrete simple activity held in a quiet setting can offer a productive, calming focus which can help a person calm down and behave more appropriately.
4. Help the **other group members** make sense of the behaviour, contain and manage it. They may need to be given some reassurance and a few ideas about how to respond. For example, as leader of an activity group, you might suggest others carry on with their tasks while you work with the individual. Alternatively, members might need to be told not to get caught up in bizarre talk and collude with delusional material. Sometimes it is intriguing to see that a person's bizarre or disruptive behaviour may be a way of expressing and reflecting tensions within the group. For an illustration of this see the Theory into Practice box below. With calm, gentle handling and a supportive group atmosphere, the behaviour may be contained.

THEORY INTO PRACTICE

Handling disruptive behaviour

Four people were working together to prepare for living with each other in a group home. They were all chronically institutionalized, having remained within the hospital system for many years. The patients were functioning at a low but fairly stable level with the exception of Martin, whose delusions had never been entirely suppressed by medication.

During one training session, Martin talked with great pressure, incoherently for 2 full minutes about spy rings, sabotage and secret codes being communicated through the water pipes. Martin seemed to become increasingly agitated. The therapist was eventually able to interrupt Martin's flow of words, gently saying, 'I'm not sure I've understood all that you're saying Martin, but I can see how upsetting it is and how worried you are'. The therapist then offered Martin the opportunity either to stay with the group activity or return to the ward. Looking somewhat calmer, Martin elected to stay.

The therapist then addressed what she saw was an underlying anxiety in the group which Martin seemed to be expressing. 'You know Martin has told us he is feeling worried at the moment. I think everyone in the group is a bit worried at this time especially about living in the group house next month. I think it would be good to spend a bit of time today looking at this area. What things are you going to find most difficult next month do you think?'

THE SILENT GROUP

The extent to which a silent group is a problem depends on the group. Fifteen minutes of silence may be acceptable in one group and a nightmare for another. Think about the following silences: which are problematic?

a) In an activity group, the atmosphere is relaxed and comfortable, and group members are absorbed in their tasks.
b) In a directive, teaching session, the leader asks the group a question. No one responds.
c) In a group discussion activity, the discussion falters and the group lapses into silence and members withdraw.

d) In a drama type group the leader asks members to do a
   certain role play activity and no one moves to carry it out.
e) In a psychotherapy group the atmosphere is tense and
   emotionally charged. Members remain silent for 20 minutes
   and responses vary – some occasionally giggle with each
   other, others look deep in thought, and others look disengaged, thinking of other things.

The situation in a) is clearly not a problem as members are
working cooperatively in a companionable silence. Although
the teacher in b) is likely to feel uncertain and tense, the silence
of the group members may mean they are thinking about how
to respond. It is more of a problem if the group is usually silent,
thus signalling their non-involvement, boredom or apathy.
The silence within the group discussion c) may be a natural
response to having run out of things to say or may reflect
either passivity or resistance to the activity or therapist. The
drama situation of d) is one we all dread, particularly as in-
experienced group therapists. By not immediately participating
with enthusiasm, the group members are signalling their
uncertainty (either confusion about directions or feeling
emotionally threatened) about the task. This is only a problem
if a route through cannot be negotiated. The psychotherapy
situation e) is a different order of silence. It is bound to be
extremely tense for all concerned and often indicates a lack of
trust where members are holding back what they might say as
they feel unable to share their stronger feelings. The silence
itself then becomes emotionally charged and emotions can
escalate with members being increasingly confused, resentful, threatened and emotionally blocked about sharing their
feelings.
   In any group we need to assess carefully the line between
positive silence where the group members are reflective and
working constructively, and negative silences. In general
negative silences occur in activity groups when members feel
bored, apathetic or are somehow resisting the activity. The
psychotherapy type group silence is invariably a demonstration
of members either not feeling engaged with the group or
overwhelmed by emotions. The silence, in either case, is a
defence.

Problem-solving ideas

1. As a general rule, regardless of the type of group, the leader should probably **wait** before intervening to break a silence. This allows the group an extra opportunity to take responsibility to sort out the situation. By rescuing the group too soon, the leader can give a message that the members are not able to handle it themselves.

2. Group leaders should also examine their **own feelings** and ask 'What is bothering me about the silence? Am I trying to push members to talk too soon to benefit my own needs?' We need to be able to handle our responses to silences, by staying calm and using the silence constructively.

3. If group members are resistant to becoming involved in an activity it may need to be **put on hold** temporarily. Get the group to reflect on their own needs and responses. The leader might say 'It seems I've lost you and you are not keen on this activity. Let's backtrack a bit and think about why we are doing this'.

4. In a psychotherapy group it is important to **allow the silence** to occur and not rescue the group from the tense feelings it will undoubtedly be experiencing. Nichols and Jenkinson (1991, p 108) advises the therapist to intervene only 'when you think that the essential safety is at risk for some members or when you feel that the silence is for negative reasons, is going nowhere, and could be turned into a useful opportunity'. Some useful questions we can pose as leaders when we want to intervene without directing are: 'How useful are people finding this silence?'; 'It seems quite difficult to speak having had this long silence. What have people been thinking but finding it difficult to say?'; 'I'm not sure what this silence is about. Is it thoughtful and comfortable or tense and difficult?'; I'm beginning to feel rather tense with this silence, are others feeling the same?'

THE APATHETIC GROUP

The apathetic, non-responsive group often poses particular problems for occupational therapists as the essence of our brand of therapy is to get people to be active and do things. In an apathetic group people are negative, unduly critical or passive, and lack the motivation to be involved in the treatment. Moreover, the energy and spontaneity of a group is diminished as apathetic feelings escalate and infect everyone (even the leader is not immune!). The apathy can then manifest in different ways, from non-participation to people wanting to leave the group or not attend in the first place.

Groups become apathetic for a variety of reasons. Members may be bored by the activity, under-stimulated by the environment or they may simply feel tired. Members may lack drive and motivation for longer term reasons caused by their illness, medication or social situation. Individuals' non-participation may express an unwillingness to be involved. If forced to attend a group against their will, why not opt out of the session itself? Finally, at a deeper level, the members may feel threatened by the group and withdraw as a defence mechanism. The apparently 'bored' behaviour in fact hides underlying 'churned-up' feelings.

Problem-solving ideas

Strategies to handle apathetic group members need to link directly to the source of the problem.

1. **Change the activity**. Can the activity be made more interesting? Introducing an element of challenge, humour or competition can raise interest. If the activity is too dull, maybe it should be dropped altogether! Can the environment be made more stimulating by introducing background noise, colour and movement?
2. Take a closer look at each individual's **problem of volition** (Kielhofner, 1985). One person may be reluctant to become involved because he or she fears failure or feels unable to carry out the task. Another individual may not feel the activity is sufficiently meaningful or fits in with his or her values. Others may need outside pressure and encouragement to overcome inertia.
3. The **policy** for group attendance should be reviewed. Ideally members should not be forced to attend and if they wish to leave it should be accepted. But occasionally, it is appropriate to encourage people to stay with the group, particularly if an issue needs to be resolved, or if the group activity would be overly disrupted by individuals leaving.

4. If the apathy is a symptom of tension and avoidance in the group as a whole, more effort needs to go into building up **trust and cohesion**. Either underlying stresses can be explored or positive group building exercises can be introduced.

5. Finally, as leaders we should examine our **own behaviour**. Are we being too active ourselves, thereby creating passive members? Are our expectations of levels of interest reasonable and realistic? Alternatively, is our own lack of commitment and interest being picked up by the group members? If we are not motivated how are we to facilitate others?

A GROUP IN CONFLICT

A group in conflict can manifest in complex ways. Anger may be expressed between group members or towards the leader. Alternatively, the group may fragment into destructive, competing cliques. The anger may be expressed in an open or a disguised manner – perhaps revealing itself in apathetic or sabotaging behaviour and undermining comments. Conflict is also reflected in subtle ways such as when a group is non-productive and members are somehow 'stuck', unable to reach agreement or work together.

Any conflict can be potentially difficult, even dangerous, as aggression can escalate and individuals get hurt. Group cohesion may be destroyed as people feel threatened and lack trust in each other. Not all conflict is negative, however, as a healthy 'performing' group is one where members feel safe enough to express their tension and can disagree constructively.

The source of conflict is often difficult to pinpoint, as a combination of factors may be involved. Individuals hit out in anger when offended, threatened or pushed in a sensitive area. Alternatively, members may be angry at the group – its aims, methods, direction. They may feel frustrated with the activity (for instance it may be too difficult), thereby creating tension. Commonly, members will feel angry with the leader – a complex process which may involve transference, competition for the leadership, or simply frustration at perceiving the leader's approach to be inadequate.

Problem-solving ideas

In many ways all the problems and problem-solving ideas discussed previously can be applied to dealing with a group in conflict. The conflict may manifest in silent or apathetic behaviour, for instance. The suggestions offered below could be used in addition to the strategies outlined earlier.

1. Our natural temptation when faced with conflict in a group is to rush in and dampen the expression – don't. First of all, it may be a **positive** 'storming' process for the group where members are being constructively honest with each other. Secondly, the members may be able to handle the situation themselves. By intervening you give the message that you have to sort things out, thereby creating dependency.
2. Encourage the **constructive expression** of the negative feelings and explore what the conflict is about. Only control the expression if it threatens the group task or makes the group feel unsafe.
3. If conflict erupts between **individuals**, it may be necessary to take them on one side to discuss the difficulty and then give responsibility to them to handle the situation more positively. Alternatively, the conflict may be brought to the **group** as a whole and discussed in terms of how the group cohesion is being threatened.
4. If tensions are being created by the **group activity** it may be necessary to modify it, for instance, inject some humour or make it easier to do. After the conflict the group may need some gentle, soothing activities or team-building exercises for group cohesion.
5. When **destructive sub-groups** emerge, we can do one of two things. We could open up discussion in the group about the dynamics and point out the negative effects. We might also restructure the group activities to encourage different sub-groupings, for instance breaking up the cliques and encouraging different members to partner each other.
6. Finally, as leaders we should examine our **own approach** carefully. Is the hostility a result of member's frustration with our leadership? Are they signalling that their needs are not being met? It is hard not to be defensive, but the group will appreciate your efforts to respond to their feedback. In

the end we might just have to put up with a certain amount of 'flack' – displaced anger goes with the territory!

This chapter has explored a range of group problems and problem-solving strategies. We have seen how the problems often reflect complex, underlying dynamics, namely, how: a) an individual can both reflect and create problems in the group as a whole, as seen with the distressed member; b) the group in turn, can subtly encourage a problem behaviour in an individual, as the example of the over-dominant member showed; c) behaviours are often interlinked, as demonstrated by members who are simultaneously silent, apathetic and angry.

Different problem-solving strategies were suggested which placed their focus either on working with **individual** members or the **group as a whole**. Equally, changes in the group **activity**, **environment** or **leadership style** were recommended.

One final point – all of us experience problems in and with groups. As leaders, sometimes we get it wrong and sometimes, right. The first step to handling any problem is to recognize that, as leaders, it is not our sole responsibility. We have neither fully created the problem, nor are we fully responsible for curing it. The group as a whole should realize their role in creating and maintaining a problem, and they should be given the chance to work out their own solutions.

8

Recording, reporting, evaluation

It may be tempting to feel that our work is done when our group activity has ended. In fact three more tasks await our attention. We need to **record** what occurred in the group, **report** these results and then **evaluate** the processes and outcomes. These three tasks are separate but interlinked. Clear record keeping aids reporting and much of what we select to report shapes and is shaped by our evaluations.

This chapter discusses why and how we might record, report on and evaluate groupwork. The message it seeks to emphasize is that these processes are an essential part of running a group. In doing this, it offers a number of practical examples of each of these aspects – more to give an opportunity for reflective comparison than as a model of how it should be done.

RECORDING

Why keep records?

Many of us seem to find record keeping difficult and tedious, so we avoid doing it. To help us overcome this reluctance it is worth thinking through why recording is an important process. We need a record of our group sessions for a number of reasons:

1. to **provide a record** of what happened, for both legal reasons and so that other staff who are absent from the session can catch up.
2. to offer a **de-briefing** opportunity where we can clarify our thoughts and express feelings.

3. to **improve our own understanding** of the group. For example, as part of our professional growth, it can be instructive to study the evolving dynamics of a group and relate this to theoretical knowledge.
4. to **develop professional skills** of observation and reflective critical thinking.
5. to **monitor progress** and help review our own performance and the group process as part of evaluation.
6. to **aid planning** subsequent sessions, for instance, reviewing comments made about previously recorded exercises can give useful ideas for the future.
7. to form the basis of official **written reports** as required.
8. to provide data for future **research**.

Each of these above points is in itself sufficient reason to write up sessions carefully. In combination, they show why good record keeping is essential.

How to keep records?

The method of record keeping needs to be established during the planning stage of a group. Decisions that might need to be made include: Who will write up the group? What format should it take? What information is needed? Who will have access to it?

Notes should be written as soon after the session as possible. It is easy to forget or distort what happened in a group, particularly when we are running several groups regularly. If you find that getting the notes written up is a problem, it may well be that you are trying to write up too much and being too ambitious about what to record. It is better to note down who attended and a few significant events, but have something written immediately, than it is to procrastinate for days and write pages. In other words, it is better to write a limited amount down immediately, than a lot later when information may be distorted. If it is difficult to write up the notes immediately after the session, try to set some time aside later in the day. If this is a problem, then perhaps the group session itself should be shortened to ensure some recording time. Adequate time to write up notes needs to be found and it should be planned as the group itself is planned.

Where there is more than one leader, it can be helpful for each of the therapists to jot down their own impressions before coming together to share their ideas. Not only is this a useful exercise to remind us about the subjectivity of our observations, it is also an invaluable opportunity to expand our perspective of what occurred in the group. To illustrate this, consider the similarities and differences of the descriptions given below where two therapists describe the same group.

It may be relevant for the group members to know what kind of record is being kept. Some leaders feel uncomfortable with this notion and consider that the patient's or client's behaviour will be unduly affected, for instance, becoming more inhibited. I would argue for a more open policy as I believe the members have a right to know and that any inhibitions which

---

Cooking group – Sarah's notes

General: The cooking group felt tense from the start (probably a result of ward tensions the night before). But also, members were excited over cooking the meal for the unit tonight.

Decision-making phase: Majority agreed to cook an Italian meal and to be guided by Mario. Patricia was annoyed, having voted for Chinese.

Cooking phase: Bill took on role as organizer and everyone followed his lead except Patricia, who seemed to resent the instruction. Mario patiently taught members, showing them how to carry out the different recipes. Tense atmosphere eased as members got involved. Half-way through I (Sarah) challenged Patricia saying she was being negative and working against the group. She exploded – threw the bowl towards me and shouted that she didn't need me to get at her as well and this was a stupid group. She stormed out and Denise went out to speak with her. The group was a bit shaken but also seemed relieved. Rest of session was productive, good humoured and uneventful.

Evaluation: Productive group. Initially tense not helped by Patricia who tended to be negative, complaining and worked against the group. The group worked well together after she stormed out. (?)Patricia's level of group affiliation? (?)Is she being scapegoated?

Cooking group – Denise's notes

0–10 min
Group tense from start about performing tonight (?) Bill took leadership role facilitating decision to cook Italian. Mario instructed members in recipes. Bill made some digs at Patricia who was tense and irritable, and (?) expressing anxiety on behalf of the group.

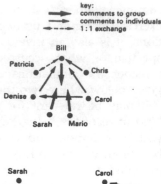

key:
comments to group
comments to individuals
1:1 exchange

Bill
Patricia
Chris
Denise
Carol
Sarah
Mario

10–45 min
Group split into sub-groups. Mario floated and taught people. Bill, Sarah and Chris worked well with laughter. Carol, Denise, Patricia quieter. Patricia a little left out. Bill and Patricia continued under breath comments. (?) Bill needling her (?)

Sarah
Carol
Denise
Chris
Bill
Mario
Patricia

45 min
Pat smashed up cooking bowl, shouted at Sarah who had made the comment that Patricia was being negative. She then stormed out, I followed for individual session (see attached notes).

do arise will not be sustained once trust develops. Even if the patients or clients do keep things secret or behave differently when they are conscious of being monitored they are still likely to participate and bring up some relevant material on which to work.

So far, I have referred to the process of record keeping in terms of writing-up a session. It is of course possible to use other methods, namely, **audio- or video-taping**. There are a number of **advantages** of taping a group session, particularly video-taping. It can be highly informative, as we are able to re-play it, examine processes more carefully and objectively, and we can be more sure of having an accurate record of the proceedings. In addition, having a video record can be highly instructive when used during supervision sessions. Lastly, the process of videoing a session can be invaluable within the group, for instance, to allow group members to observe their own behaviour.

The **disadvantages** of such a method of record keeping are firstly, that it is time-consuming to re-play and you still need to write up some notes as well. However, simply sampling bits of a session can be illuminating, and using the recording selectively cuts down on time. Secondly, some therapists are reluctant to use a tape in a group because of their own inexperience, shyness or fears that it will inhibit the members. These reasons may be valid, but need to be worked through and balanced against the value of having such an accurate record of events. Finally, if members are reluctant to be videoed, then there are two courses of action: either to respect their wishes; or to allow them more time to get used to the technology – playing around with filming in a fun sort of way can greatly ease feelings of self-consciousness.

Types of records

What records we keep depends on unit practice, the group's purpose, how the records are to be used and what the people reading the records need to know. In practice, we are likely to need to keep three different types of records or some combination of these.

Factual records. These record who attends the group, for how long, the date, type and aim of session, descriptions of activities carried out and any relevant information about individuals.

Records on individuals. In some units information of individual's performance and progress may be the only record kept. This type of information is most relevant for task and activity groups. Such records can be unstructured and simply involve comments being written in the patient's or client's notes or Kardex. Structured records are extensions of specific assessments where we might carry out a behaviour count (for example, noting the number of times a patient has to hand wash in an art session) or use a relevant rating scale (such as for assessing cognitive function). Tables 8.1 and 8.2 offer two

Table 8.1 Participation record

Group participation assessment						
Behaviour	Individual names					
	Dick	Terry	Julie	Jane	Ben	Sally
Encourages						
Agrees						
Provides humour						
Suggests						
Asks questions						
Answers questions						
Instructs						
Analyses						
Depreciates self						
Is aggressive						
Is self-assertive						
Withdraws						

Instructions: note number of occasions each behaviour is observed.

different forms to record individual performance. Table 8.3 represents a form which notes both individual performance and is a group record. Note how these types of forms help the leader or recorder to focus attention on specific points to observe in the group.

Process analysis. It is often important to record the dynamics of what occurs in a group and why, particularly for communication and psychotherapy groups. The following aspects could be explored: roles individuals play; communication patterns (quantity and quality); sub-groupings, alliances and relation-

Table 8.2 Self-rating record

Self-rating form – Project Group		

Name: ....   Ward: ....

Week ending: ....

Rating scale: 1 = very difficult; 2 = difficult; 3 = average; 4 = good; 5 = no problem.

	Rating	*Comments*
1. Concentrate on the task activity for one hour		
2. Share equipment/materials with other group members		
3. Get on with other people in group		
4. Talk with other people in group		
5. Appreciate the needs and problems of other group members		
6. Appreciate my own needs and difficulties in the group		

My aim for next week is:

ships; mood and tempo; evolving themes; leader's role, interventions, reactions. (An example of process analysis is given in Theory into Practice, p 193–4)

REPORTING

Why report?

Anyone working within a team will recognize the importance of good communication and liaison. As **therapists**, we rou-

Table 8.3 Group and individual performance record

Activity group ———————————————— Date ————

Topics covered/materials used

———————————————————————————————————

———————————————————————————————————

Patient's names	Motivation/ involvement	Concentration	Orientation/ memory	Mood	Interaction

Rating: 0 = no problem; 1 = some problem; 2 = severe problem.

———————————————————————————————————

Comments on individual behaviour

———————————————————————————————————

———————————————————————————————————

Comments on group as whole

———————————————————————————————————

———————————————————————————————————

Therapist role

———————————————————————————————————

———————————————————————————————————

Evaluation (strengths/weaknesses)

———————————————————————————————————

———————————————————————————————————

Future sessions – ideas

———————————————————————————————————

———————————————————————————————————

tinely give reports on patients and clients in order to discuss their needs and progress. As **groupworkers**, there are some other more specific reasons why we need to report on the groups we run.

1. Other staff can give helpful feedback on how they see the patient's or client's behaviour and reactions to the group. They may also be able to contribute their own experiences with the person and give ideas and constructive criticism about the group.
2. If other staff are aware of the group they are in a better position to: a) make more appropriate referrals, b) remind patients or clients to go to the group as appropriate, and c) respect the group times (for instance, not to ask to see a patient during those times). We also need to talk about our group as a public relations exercise, in order to help others

---

THEORY INTO PRACTICE

Sample process analysis

Present: Ron, Mark, Chris, Steve, Ruth, Daisy, myself.
Content: A cohesive group, no sub-grouping. Daisy facilitated the group by saying Karen was not coming back and trying to access everyone's feelings about this. Everyone felt sad for Karen but very little other emotion was expressed – as the group progressed other issues were raised surrounding the theme of bereavement and anger. We worked through these issues and at the end of the group Daisy related it back to Karen which had some effect with people beginning to acknowledge feelings and inter-relate issues.

1. Mark – main emphasis of group on him. He talked primarily about his anger being like a volcano inside and how it comes out every so often, out of control. He said he doesn't know why he feels this. Mark also talked about having no feelings about his father's death – feeling indifferent. In response, the group tried to show him he had a lot of anger inside which had built up over the years because he was not expressing himself. Mark denied this emphatically and could not see it.

2. Steve also shared quite a bit, saying how important it was to let off angry feelings – though he never actually expressed emotion himself. He talked in distant advisory terms. I confronted him which made him angry in turn and he was able to express some anger at the end about Karen leaving.
3. Ron was supportive and talked of feeling angry with his parents and wishing he had been able to tell them before their death. He felt relieved at off-loading in the group.
4. My intervention pointing out three levels of working through anger: a) recognizing it, b) expressing it, c) expressing it to the person concerned. Mark is at stage a) and trying to run to c) as he has expressed anger to his mother yet denies any to his father. Ron has reached b). Steve is moving from a) to b).

Key themes: working through anger and bereavement seen in relation to Karen leaving. Difficulties of expressing true emotion, particularly anger.
Facilitators' role: Daisy drew links with the themes of working through anger and bereavement about Karen. I felt more comfortable this week and felt good about my challenging interventions.

better understand our role and contribution to the treatment team.

3. A number of situations require us to be very clear and precise in our communications with each other in the team. Some typical examples where liaison is vital are: when a patient or client is using the situation inappropriately and playing off one therapist against another; when therapists are at cross purposes in different groups, thereby confusing the patient or client; when problems, about which the group therapist is unaware, arise after the group session (for example, a patient regularly being aggressive).

How to report?

Reports on a group can be written or verbal, informal or formal. Whichever method is chosen, the channels of communication should be established beforehand. For instance, feedback time needs to be set aside in advance or the group leader may agree to write a summary report at the end of the set of sessions.

Formal, written reports are rarely provided about a group but may be requested on an individual. Such a report needs to provide succinct statements about aims of treatment, the individual's performance and recommendations for future actions.

The group itself may be best reported verbally (formal or informal). **Verbal reports** allow discussion where the reporter can gain support as well as give information. Whittaker (1986, p 135) advises groupworkers to '... communicate both one's pleasure and one's disappointments: the exciting, productive sessions as well as the difficult ones. Accurate, honest communications rather than selective and hence misleading reports are most likely to contribute to ... realistic views about groups.'

Table 8.4 Types of reports

Report to	Level and content	Aims
other OTs who have referred the clients to the group	extensive feedback at the end of each session; focus on individual's progress	to give feedback on individual's performance and to evaluate aims and treatment methods
multi-disciplinary team	brief summary evaluation at end of 12 week group	professional exchange of ideas
supervisor and group leaders	in-depth analysis of process and leader's role	to understand group dynamics and improve leader's performance
outside GP	brief written report indicating individual's current status	to report on individual's progress
managers	written evaluation of benefits of group	to argue the case for more resources to repeat the group

The **level and content** of any report can vary depending on the context, needs of team members involved and the aims of the report. Table 8.4 lays out a variety of situations where we might encounter reports.

As a final point, the group members have a right (morally if not legally*) to know what type of information is being shared with whom. Tempting as it is to assure patients or clients that the group will be 'confidential', we can rarely guarantee it in practice. We work within a team where some material has to be shared. It is therefore a misplaced way of trying to build trust. Invariably, some of the confidential material will be fed back to the patient or client from another source, thereby destroying any trust permanently. My usual tactic in a group is to say 'Anything that happens in this group will be kept in total confidence by the team. If anything seems particularly relevant to your treatment, I will share it with the other team members who need to know'. I might then follow this up by asking for a 'group contract of confidentiality' where they avoid sharing material with outsiders. This is normally agreed and does much to promote respect for, and trust in, the group.

EVALUATION

It is our professional responsibility to evaluate our work. Some of us may be unsure how to translate this into practice. It is easy to become overwhelmed with the range of processes and problems to be evaluated. For one thing, not only do we monitor individual's progress, we also have to evaluate overall group processes and their effectiveness. Further, it can be hard to decide which of the many evaluation tools to use. This section explores evaluation at two levels. First the basic questions of why?, what?, how? and when? we evaluate groups will be answered. Then a final section places special emphasis on the research process as a form of evaluation and a selection of research findings relevant to occupational therapy groups are presented.

---

*The current legal position in the United Kingdom is that patients and clients have freedom of access to their treatment notes.

Evaluation of a group

Why evaluate?

There are at least three good reasons why we should evaluate our groupwork.

1. To establish whether or not the patients or clients are benefiting from this type of therapy – pre-and post-group assessment results can (and should) be compared to **measure progress**.
2. To aid future group **planning** – careful analysis of what has occurred in a group can help to clarify our understanding of what we should try to achieve in future groups and how they should be approached.
3. To monitor and **improve our own skills** – evaluation of our interventions will aid our future performance and in the process sharpen our skills of observation and understanding.

What to evaluate

The decision about what to evaluate is a hard one as groups involve many complex processes. Five different, but inter-linked elements need to be examined, though depending on the type of group under scrutiny, some will be more relevant than others.

i) **Group processes and interactions** – we can examine how the group operated as a whole. What roles did members play? How did they interact? What norms and themes dominated? How much cohesion and trust developed?
ii) **Individual member's performance** – often, we need to assess the performance of each of the members separately and monitor progress in behaviour, feelings or skills. Individuals may have their own treatment objectives, the outcomes of which need to be evaluated. Note that individuals might also evaluate themselves.
iii) **Activity or medium** – was the selected activity or treatment medium suitable? Was it structured and paced appropriately? What was the impact on the environment? How did members respond? How might it be graded or adapted in the future?

iv) **Own performance as leader** – self-appraisal can be hard to do. Some relevant questions to pose are: Was what I said/did helpful? Was my approach appropriate? Was I at risk of getting caught up in the group dynamics? How did I feel? This last question is often the most revealing.

v) **Co-leaders' performance** – evaluating how two or more leaders operate and interact together is as important as evaluating each leader's behaviour. The partners might ask: Did we work together? How were we being used by the group? What styles of leadership did we adopt and did they mesh? How similar are our perceptions of the group? Note that the group members might also participate in this evaluation.

How to evaluate

The many evaluation methods available can be placed along a continuum, moving from **objective**, systematic, analytical measures through to **subjective**, impressionistic accounts (see Figure 8.1). At one end of this spectrum, evaluation takes place against set criteria, while at the other end, emotional reactions are explored.

Some group leaders may rely on only one method while others may use several of them. The type of group will often determine which evaluation method needs to be used. On the one hand, a psychotherapy group will need to evaluate the group through members sharing their feelings about it plus the therapists' own observation, analysis and discussion. By contrast, a social skills training group is likely to find it more useful to evaluate outcomes by comparing pre-group with post-group measurements of social behaviour. External factors can also play a part, shaping the method adopted. Unit policy may demand the use of a standard method or some

Measuring achievement against behavioural objectives	Observation and analysis of verbal and non-verbal group content	Observation and analysis of group dynamics	Structured feedback (e.g. One thing I have gained)	Discussion of feelings and impressions

Figure 8.1 Continuum of objective/subjective evaluation methods.

THEORY INTO PRACTICE

Operationalizing goals to act as objective criteria for
evaluation

AIMS/GOALS	OBSERVATION
improve social interaction	quantity and quality of interaction using Bales
improve awareness of others' needs	unprompted sharing of materials
increase group cohesion	members express a desire to be in the group

---

form of hard evidence and objective measure of a group's
effectiveness.

There are many evaluation forms available to occupational
therapists which help us record and analyse relevant data.
Consider the sample forms on the following pages (Tables 8.5,
8.6, 8.7). What are their strengths and weaknesses? In what
situations might they be best employed? Are there elements
from several examples which could be combined into another
form?

When to evaluate

Evaluating may be wrongly perceived as a process which only
occurs at the end of a group and is therefore only often written
up as an afterthought or postscript. In fact, the process is an
integral part of an on-going group and needs to occur as part of
every phase.

First, in the **planning phase**, when goals, methods and
activities are being established, the evaluation criteria is also
being laid down. If the goals for the group are to promote
interaction and share materials, for example, one criterion of
evaluation needs to relate to the degree that members are able
to share by the end of the group session.

Second, **during the group session**, we need to monitor
constantly the activities and group processes and adapt the
environment in response to our on-going evaluations. For
instance, we may observe one member being excluded and

Table 8.5 Assertion training course evaluation

Name: ....   Date: ....

Please rate each aspect of the course with a number from 1 to 10
(1 = not useful experience, 10 = very useful experience). Also,
please write any comments to back up your rating and give
suggestions for the future.

Introduction to group _____   _____

_____

Warm-up/down games _____   _____

_____

Communication exercises _____   _____

_____

Modelled role-plays _____   _____

_____

Role plays _____   _____

_____

Feedback/criticism _____   _____

_____

Discussion _____   _____

_____

Theory _____   _____

_____

Goal-setting _____   _____

_____

Group conclusion _____   _____

_____

Overall comments _____

_____

_____

_____

Table 8.6 General group evaluation

We would appreciate your ideas and comments about the group to help us evaluate how it has gone. Knowing what aspects have worked well (and which didn't) will also aid our future planning. Please complete the following sentences to reflect **your** experience of the group.

1. The most enjoyable aspects of the group were

_____

_____

_____

2. The least enjoyable aspects of the group were

_____

_____

_____

3. The most beneficial aspects of the groups were

_____

_____

_____

4. The group could be improved by

_____

_____

Any other comments/suggestions:

Thank you for your cooperation and time in filling out this form.

so take steps to shift the focus of the group. We could also encourage group members to air their views, needs and ideas during a group, and then modify the activity in response to their feedback.

Third, towards the **end of a session** we often ask members how they experienced the group activity. The members' perspectives are usually illuminating. The process of group evaluation also encourages members to be more involved in the group's development.

Fourth, **after the group**, we will need to review what has

Table 8.7 Group process evaluation

A. Group goals
   1. No goals
   2. Some goals or goals slightly confused
   3. Goals very clear
   Comments:

B. Quantity/quality of work accomplished
   1. No work accomplished
   2. Average accomplishments
   3. Great deal of quality work accomplished
   Comments:

C. Group atmosphere
   1. Hostile, uncomfortable, negative
   2. Average, atmosphere reasonable
   3. Highly supportive, cooperative, warm
   Comments:

D. Group cohesion/trust
   1. Group fragmented or lacking in trust
   2. Average
   3. Strong sense of belonging and trust
   Comments:

E. Participation
   1. Limited and uneven, group participation/involvement
   2. Average participation involvement
   3. A great deal of participation/involvement
   Comments:

F. Sensitivity
   1. Group members self-absorbed, insensitive, not listening
   2. Average sensitivity, some less, some more
   3. Outstanding sensitivity, listening, empathy
   Comments:

G. Group decisions
   1. No decisions or decisions made by few
   2. Majority decisions accepted
   3. Full participation and tested consensus
   Comments:

H. Leadership
   1. Poor
   2. Average or slightly uneven
   3. Good, attentive, facilitative
   Comments:

occurred and appraise both members' performances and the functioning of the group as a whole.

Fifth, at the **end of the group series**, we will need to reflect on the benefits and limitations of the group programme. Which aspects proved most effective? Which elements proved counter-productive? For example, we might find that while the number of planned sessions allowed relationships to be built up, they did not give adequate opportunity to conclude the groupwork.

THEORY INTO PRACTICE

Encouraging group involvement in evaluation

AT THE START: If you are expecting group members to participate in the process of giving feedback and evaluation, they need to be involved and thinking at an early stage. As the group begins, ensure group goals and expectations are clear, as this establishes the baseline for future evaluation.

Some example methods:

a) 'Want–don't want' exercise – pairs or small groups brainstorm what they want and don't want from the group. These are then matched up with the leader's hopes, expectations and fears. The answers are preserved on a flipchart which can be referred to at the end of the group in order to evaluate the extent that needs were met.

b) 'Goal-sabotage' exercise – each individual states at least one goal for attending the group and acknowledges one way he or she might sabotage any gains or be prevented from achieving the goal. This exercise encourages individuals to take responsibility for their growth.

c) Use of an evaluation form – give each group member a copy of the group evaluation form to be used at the end of the group series. Ask the members to be aware of the categories and to fill it out as they go along, as this ensures important details are not forgotten from session to session. This exercise signals the expectation that members contribute to the group's evaluation.

DURING THE GROUP: As the group develops, encourage members to reflect on their experience regularly and to give on-the-spot feedback. This sets an open, responsive tone and demonstrates that you value, and will respond to their opinions.

Some example methods:

a) Discussion – regularly ask members for their reactions to the group and activity.
b) Scoring – at the end of an exercise, game or role-play, ask the group members to hold up their fingers to give a score as appropriate. One finger could mean 'needs changing', three fingers could mean 'very good', This type of scoring can be a quick, useful way to rate an individual's role play performance and is often experienced as less threatening than receiving comments as it is non-verbal and occurs amongst all the members simultaneously.

AFTER THE GROUP: The time for the most focused evaluation is at the end of a group session or group series. At an informal level, members are likely to exchange comments. At a more formal level, members may be asked specific questions or may even be required to fill out an evaluation form.

Some example methods:

a) Structured feedback – each member shares two things he or she has 'gained' from the group, one thing 'not liked' and one 'suggestion' for the future. This provides a comprehensive feedback and helps the group end on a constructive note.
b) Evaluation form – the ritual of written feedback can be a valuable supplement to verbal comments. It provides a concrete record and allows quieter members to have their say.

RESEARCH

So far this chapter has focused on the evaluation of specific groups. What about evaluation of groups in general? What groups do we run? How effective are they? Is one type of group better than another? What proof is there? Here we come into the province of research and what it might offer. This section explores the process of research; first by discussing its value and limitations, and then by offering some actual examples of research on groupwork.

Value and limitations

Research is necessary to help us **understand** the group process better. Specifically, we need to understand how a group operates, what effects the group process, and how the process in turn, effects the group members. Knowing what makes a group work assists us to be more **effective** in our therapeutic use of it. We are then in a position to know what treatment format to select to meet our therapeutic aims and we will have a better understanding of which problems we can treat in a group and how. We will also have solid evidence to back up our professional assumptions and intuition.

In the current competitive climate, we are becoming increasingly aware of the need to evaluate, and even **justify**, our work. Research can validate the role of particular kinds of groupwork. We might at the same time, validate the contribution of occupational therapy within an overall treatment programme.

Having stressed the importance of doing research on occupational therapy groupwork, I do not underestimate the difficulties involved. Potential researchers are confronted with two main barriers. One is the current **pool of literature**, which is hard to interpret and link to occupational therapy. A lot of research on groups has been done, but findings are often contradictory and the diversity of groups and outcomes studied can be confusing. Moreover, very little of the research relates directly to occupational therapy practice. Many of the findings pertaining to psychotherapy may have relevance for occupational therapy, but links need to be made and generalizations from one field to another are not necessarily valid. In all, we have few studies which can guide us in future group practice and research.

A second barrier to research is that groups are both notoriously difficult to study and raise all sorts of **methodological problems**. By definition, group processes are multiple and complex and this creates difficulties for researchers who are trying to control variables and disentangle effects. Further, no two groups are identical and this makes it hard to compare groups, or even, to replicate studies.

Whilst hard evidence in the form of objective, structured empirical research may be difficult to come by, much informal observation exists. Nichols and Jenkinson (1991, p 21) pick up this point when they assert, 'The sheer weight of "clinical" evidence . . . and consumer feedback is enormous and more than enough to remove doubts about the essential issue, namely that helping groups are an effective, credible, and worthwhile resource in giving care.' As a profession we need to tap the knowledge and experience which undoubtedly exists and build our pool of resources.

Some research examples

Read over the examples of groupwork research below. The list is highly selective, but is in my view, representative of the current state of the art. All the examples have particular relevance to occupational therapy. Consider their methods and findings. Do these findings help increase our understanding of groupwork, its application and value? Do they spark off an interest in you and give you some ideas to pursue in your own research?

Survey method

A good example of descriptive surveys is one carried out by Duncombe and Howe (1985) who surveyed 200 occupational therapists (in all specialities) in the United States to determine their use of groups. Sixty per cent of the therapists said they used groupwork and 76% of these used activity (or activity with a verbal component) formats. The most frequently used groups were activities of daily living groups (17%), reality-oriented discussion (15.5%), sensory–motor activities (13.5%) and arts and crafts (10.5%). Most groups had more than one goal, the most common one being to increase socialization and communication.

My comment – this basic piece of research establishes some useful facts about current groupwork practice. We need to collect similar data for practice in the United Kingdom. This would be a good study to replicate on either a national or regional basis.

Controlled studies

A number of researchers have investigated the value of activity groups over talking groups, an issue which is of fundamental importance to our work as occupational therapists.

1. McDermott (1988) considered the effect of three types of group formats (task, activity-based verbal, and verbal) on interaction patterns. The Bales system of Interaction Process Analysis was used to describe the quantity and quality of interactions in a psychiatric (non-psychotic) population. The task group was found to have more positive socio-emotional communications (compliments, expressed satisfaction, joking), more interactions between members, and fewer uninvolved members. The verbal and activity-based verbal groups contained more discussion of feelings, comments to the whole group, and leader involvement. All three groups were seen to be beneficial for learning, in different ways.

My comment – this study demonstrates the value of using a task group to help decrease social isolation and promote social skills. It could be replicated with other patient and client groups, for instance, with people who are physically handicapped but mentally stable.

2. Klyczek and Mann (1986) compared different treatment programs at two psychiatric day centres. One offered twice as much psychotherapy as activity, the other offered twice as much activity as psychotherapy. The activity oriented program was found to be significantly more effective with respect to a wide range of symptoms such as, decision-making skills, use of leisure time, self-esteem and vocational adjustment. Interestingly, the activity group yielded a greater rate of relapse though the length of stay during hospitalization was shorter. Overall the findings suggest that 'activities and the process of "doing", as inherent in occupational therapy treatment, do in fact facilitate the patient's faster return to higher or more adaptive levels of functioning than do verbal therapy techniques.' (Klyczek and Mann 1986, p 610).

My comment – this type of study is crucial in validating our occupational therapy contribution and needs to be replicated in a range of hospital and community centres.

3. De-Carlo and Mann (1985) compared the effects of activity and verbal groups on psychiatric patients' (self-reported) interpersonal skills. Both groups met for eight sessions and results were compared to a control group who received normal milieu therapy. The

Interpersonal Communication Inventory was used as the pre-test and post-test measure of improvements. Results demonstrated that interpersonal skills of the activity group subjects increased significantly more than the verbal group. The fact that neither group performed significantly better than the control group may be due to the methodological limitations of this study and deserves further attention.

My comment – a strength of this study is the author's recognition of patient's or client's own perception of the benefits of group treatment. We might routinely ask similar questions when we invite group members to evaluate our groups. This data could be extended into a research project.

Some studies investigate the value of specific elements within a group treatment programme. To give a flavour of the range possible, here are three different projects:

4. Kremer, Nelson and Duncombe (1984) investigated the degree of meaning different activities held for chronic psychiatric patients. Twenty-two patients were randomly assigned to three groups: cooking, craft and sensory awareness groups. After the group activity, each patient rated its affective meaning using Osgood's Semantic differential scale. Results showed differences in meaning for each activity with cooking found to be significantly more meaningful than the others. The authors discuss the possible reasons for this, being that it is a concrete activity with a consumable end-product; it offers oral stimulation; it is age appropriate and culturally meaningful.

My comment – the model of human occupation (Kielhofner, 1985) describes the meaningfulness of activity as an important element in increasing a person's volition to be involved in activity. Investigating whether and why activities are valued would appear to be a central task for occupational therapists to do within the context of different cultures.

5. Henry, Nelson and Duncombe (1984) investigated people's affective responses to having or lacking freedom of choice in completing an activity. They also explored how those responses differed when the subjects did the activity in individual or group situations. Forty female students participated in an origami activity under four experimental conditions: a) individual-choice, b) individual-no choice, c) group-choice, d) group-no choice. Afterwards, each person rated how she felt about herself whilst participating in terms of evaluation, power and activity. Subjects in the group with no choice of activity rated themselves as feeling significantly less powerful than those with a choice.

My comment – this finding emphasizes how the presence of others (group) acts as a source of feedback and can change how we perceive ourselves. The finding supports one of our basic occupational therapy assumptions, that it is important to include members in shaping a group activity.

6. Yalom, Houts, Newell and Rank (1967) investigated specific methods of preparing patients for group psychotherapy. They compared the effectiveness of having a specific group preparatory session with simply doing a history-taking interview. Sixty patients awaiting group therapy were assigned to each condition (six groups in all). The findings show that the prepared group had a number of advantages. Firstly, the patients had more faith in therapy which in turn was seen to influence outcomes positively. Secondly, the patients were more involved and interacted more in the group.

My comment – this study investigated whether the inclusion of a particular technique helped a group be more effective. Whilst it refers to psychotherapy groups, could the findings generalize to other groups?

Qualitative studies

Many, more descriptive, studies contribute to our experiential knowledge. These studies typically describe and analyse a group process.

Blair (1979) offered a brief account of a 9 month long supportive psychotherapy group with elderly psychiatric patients. She describes key themes which arose, for instance, feelings about retirement, grief, loneliness. The author mentions the group seemed to have a 'positive binding effect for both staff and patient' (Blair, 1979 p 138), a factor which needs further exploration.

Monroe and Herron (1980) similarly describe a 1-week combined projective art and group therapy experience consisting of 12 sessions. A brief account of each session was given along with the therapeutic gains and problems (at an individual and group level) were discussed. The authors conclude that 'art sessions enable individuals to express some of their less articulate aspects of experience, while the group therapy with words enables them to clarify, to understand . . .' (Munroe and Herron, 1980, p 24).

My comment – studies like these are a good first step, documenting our daily work. Many therapists are running interesting, special groups, but the rest of the profession does not know about it. I would like to see us benefitting from a more public sharing of our work.

Literature reviews

'Armchair research' (Stewart, 1990, p 532) in the form of literature reviews offer a wide range of possibilities to investigate the current state of the art and science of groupwork.

Brady (1984) offers an in-depth review of social skills training studies. Overall, the findings suggest that modelling, practice, feedback and structured interaction are effective ways to teach social skills. The results also suggest that social skills are better learned through practising in a group rather than talking about them. The author notes some discrepancies and methodological flaws in the studies (such as failing to control for diagnosis).

Kanas (1986) reviewed 43 controlled studies on group therapy with schizophrenics. The author concluded that 'group therapy was judged to be an effective modality of treatment for schizophrenics in 67% of the inpatient studies . . . 80% of the outpatient studies. Interaction-oriented approaches were more effective than insight-oriented approaches which were found to be harmful for some schizophrenics.' (Kanas, 1986, p 339)

My comment – these reviews consider the effectiveness of particular group methods and are valuable for exploring any aspect of groupwork be it related to incidence or effectiveness. However, we need studies to review in the first place. Currently most of the literature refers to psychotherapy – the next step is to expand our occupational therapy research base.

I have been necessarily selective in presenting a range of different types of research studies. No one study alone offers a definitive account of the effectiveness of groupwork but as a growing pool of evidence, it starts to carry some weight. All of these studies can be used and need to be replicated and expanded to encompass different patient and client groups in different settings. New research also needs to minimize the methodological difficulties apparent in the past literature. Research on group treatment is, at best, an inexact science, but do not let its limitations stop us from doing the research. We have to start somewhere . . . so have **you** got some ideas?

9

Developing group leader skills

In order to learn how to lead groups, we need opportunities to practise participating in and running groups, as well as time to reflect on the process. Our training continues after we have qualified as therapists – it is our professional responsibility to keep abreast of new research and techniques in order to ensure good standards of practice. We never stop learning, no matter what level of experience we reach, and we all need continued support and guidance in helping us to develop our skills.

This concluding chapter focuses on developing group leader skills. How do we learn the skills in the first place? How can we continue to extend them? This chapter considers how learners and experienced group leaders can benefit from a combination of a) supervised practice b) observation c) experiential training.

SUPERVISED PRACTICE

The only way to acquire group leader skills is to **practise** leading groups. Alongside the practice, however, it is vital for a leader to have some **supervision**. In fact, all of us, no matter how experienced, will benefit from having a supervisor. As group leaders we all have times when we run out of ideas, or have difficult sessions, or feel confused. On the positive side, we can also get excited by our group and need to express our enthusiasm. At such times, it is valuable to have someone to go to who can offer support, guidance and feedback. The supervisor acts as mentor – an experienced and trusted advisor. This section outlines what supervision involves and then identifies some of the problems and issues which can arise within supervision.

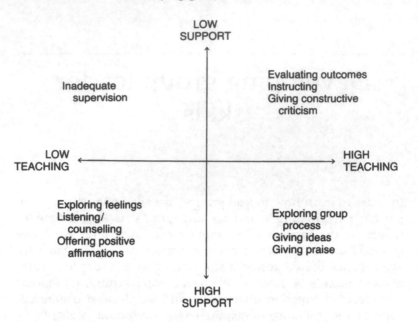

LOW
SUPPORT

Inadequate
supervision

Evaluating outcomes
Instructing
Giving constructive
criticism

LOW
TEACHING

HIGH
TEACHING

Exploring feelings
Listening/
counselling
Offering positive
affirmations

Exploring group
process
Giving ideas
Giving praise

HIGH
SUPPORT

Figure 9.1 The supervisor's role encompassing two dimensions of supervision – support and teaching.

What is supervision?

Supervision is well described in terms of how it involves two dimensions – support and teaching (see Figure 9.1). On the **support** side, the supervisor can listen and allow the group therapist to express triumphs and pleasures whilst giving support for mistakes and difficulties. On the **teaching** side, the supervisor can instruct, offer ideas and give constructive feedback. He or she should be in a position to offer a new perspective on the group which could be helpful for the group leader.

The balance of support and teaching offered in supervision will vary. Sometimes the group leader requires high levels of both, whilst at other times he or she will have a specific need for one or the other. When the group leader feels neither supported or guided, the quality of the supervision is clearly inadequate.

THEORY INTO PRACTICE

Aims of supervision

The content of a supervision session can vary according to the needs of the group leader. The supervision session could focus on either the group process or the therapist's feelings – whichever seems more relevant at the time. Consider any group that you may be leading at the moment. Which of the following aims do you most need to include in your supervision?

1. To explore and so better understand group dynamics.
2. To share ideas for activities in order to clarify the group's future direction.
3. To consider the impact of your approach on the group.
4. To extend your repertoire of ways to intervene.
5. To explore your feelings and to use the opportunity to express uncertainties about the group or how it is handled.
6. To explore co-leader relationships and any communication difficulties which arise between you.
7. To receive constructive feedback and encouragement.

A supervision session should ideally take place after – but not immediately after – each group as this gives the group therapist an opportunity to reflect on his or her performance and the group process.

This may not always be practical, for instance, when a group leader runs several, different sessions a week. In this case, a once weekly general supervision may be preferred. When trying to decide the best use of time, it may be beneficial to distinguish between activity and support groups. Leaders of support groups are likely to require more supervision opportunities due to the nature of their work than is the case with activity group leaders.

Supervision mostly occurs on a **one-to-one** basis between the group leader and the supervisor. It can also take place within a peer group discussion or with **several therapists** and one supervisor. Alternatively, a **co-supervision** arrangement may evolve when two or more leaders supervise each other.

However the supervision is structured, the key ingredient

is the relationship between the supervisor and the group leader/s. Often we do not have a choice about who acts as our supervisor. For example, the head occupational therapist may take the position automatically. This may be generally acceptable, but sometimes it is not appropriate. As group leaders, we have the right and responsibility to find a supervisor who best meets our needs. We need to have confidence in our supervisor and feel that he or she has the necessary skills to be able to listen, understand and challenge us in a positive way.

Problems and issues

Ideally, the supervisory relationship should be experienced as supportive and encouraging whilst being challenging and thought provoking. However, tensions can creep into the relationship in ways which prevent it working in a constructive manner. Four examples of problem situations which typically arise in the relationship are presented below.

1. *Pam, a group therapist, tends to operate at a superficial level in her supervision. She avoids bringing material to the session. She tries to cut the sessions short and regularly gives the message 'I don't have anything to say – everything is fine'.*

In this situation, it is the supervisory relationship which is in question. Why is Pam reluctant to share her experiences? Does she lack trust in her supervisor's responses? Does she feel too exposed and vulnerable and fears being judged? The stressfulness of being a supervisee needs to be acknowledged. Everyone feels tensions about being a learner, particularly when we make mistakes or feel that we are inadequate and failing in some way. This can become harder when we are qualified and feel we 'should' know. As supervisees, we often feel ambivalent – we want guidance and feedback, yet seek to avoid exposure.

A good tip for the supervisor is to avoid commenting on how a group should have been handled, that is to say, being critical of what occurred. It is better to focus on the here-and-now and how the group might be handled in the future. This positive, constructive approach should lessen the supervisee's stress about being judged.

2. *Ian, a group therapist, and his supervisor are at cross purposes. They view the supervision in a different light. Ian would like some guidance about how to manage the group, whilst the supervisor is interested in hearing about Ian's feelings. Ian is frustrated, and even a little threatened, by the supervisor's persistent counselling approach.*

Ideally, it is the group therapist who should set the agenda for supervision. In turn, the supervisor must try to be aware of what the group therapist needs and wants. Understandably, Ian feels frustrated and needs to ask the supervisor why there is such an emphasis on feelings.

3. *Anne, a supervisor, has too many conflicting roles in relation to Joan, the group leader. Anne has to monitor Joan's performance as well as give support. Joan is beginning to feel like 'big brother' is watching her and it is interfering with the supervisory relationship.*

Many of us are familiar with these difficulties particularly in the context of being a fieldwork supervisor of students, where we are required to straddle the roles of supporter, teacher and assessor. Sometimes the tensions are unavoidable. The above situation might be resolved by holding separate monitoring and supervision sessions. Alternatively, the roles could be split between different people. One group leader I know has a satisfactory arrangement where she goes to her peers for support, her head for teaching, and has a monthly analytically-based supervision session with a psychotherapist.

4. Very occasionally, problems within a group can be reflected in the supervision process, and vice versa. Similar issues and atmospheres can arise in both settings in quite uncanny ways. Two illustrations of this are:

a) *Julie, a therapist working in a group of demanding adolescents, found herself the focus of silent aggression and anti-authority feelings. Often group members were sullen and refused to cooperate. Julie appeared to be transferring similar feelings into her supervision in that when her supervisor offered her a suggestion about how to handle the group, she felt she was being criticized and became defensive.*

b) *John, a busy group therapist, often arrived late for or had to cancel his supervision. Eventually, the supervisor challenged*

this apparent lack of commitment and in discussion it became
clear that the group was going through a similar 'apathy phase'.
Both John and the supervisor recognized the possibility that the
group members were feeling vulnerable and threatened, and
were therefore unwilling to open up and commit themselves to
the group. On reflection, John realized the relevance of this to
his supervision.

OBSERVATION

Observing another group leader in action presents an ideal
opportunity to learn about group leadership. We can pick
up relevant techniques and model on the leader's successful
interventions, as well as gaining new ideas for activities and
exercises. We can also observe the continuum of success and
failure experienced by all group workers. Witnessing an
'expert' therapist voice anxieties or make mistakes can be
enormously comforting for the 'novice'!

As a learner, we can observe a leader leading a group in
three ways. First, it may be possible to sit in and **simply
observe** a group in action. We should observe as unobtrusively
as possible by sitting slightly away from the group. (If you
are going to do this, ensure you have the group member's
permission beforehand – they will usually agree, particularly if
you are only watching the therapist!)

Secondly, we may take part in the group activity as another
group member. This lessens possible feelings of self-consciousness in group members about being observed. This
method of **participant-observation** is widely practised by
students on fieldwork experience. Taking part in a group offers
a unique opportunity for the observer to examine group
members responses to the leader from their perspective.

THEORY INTO PRACTICE

Observing groups in order to learn prior to leading them

The length of time we observe a leader or group before we
lead one ourselves depends on: a) the type of group and
b) our level of experience as shown by Table 9.1 below.

Table 9.1 Observing before leading groups

Type of groups	Level of learner's experience	Observation time
Craft group	student occupational therapist who has experience of other craft groups	take part in the group as a member for two sessions; act as co-leader for two more sessions; then take full responsibility to plan and lead a group with the therapist present
Social skills training group	basic grade therapist with little experience of following through a long term group	act as observer/stooge member of the group for full twelve session training course; then co-lead (with an experienced leader) a similar group
Psychotherapy	experienced group therapist but limited experience of psychotherapy groups	observe an on-going psychotherapy group through one-way screen; training sessions with supervisor using video extracts; then co-lead a group with an experienced partner.

Thirdly, it can be valuable to use a **video or one-way screen** to observe a leader and group. Playing back recorded material enables us to undertake a deeper analysis of the group therapist's interventions. This method is widely adopted for family therapy and psychotherapy training.

Sometimes it is not possible to observe a group – either the technology is unavailable or the group members find observers too inhibiting. It is probable that observers would not be allowed in most occupational therapy support groups. Whilst not being able to take part in these groups is frustrating to learner groupworkers, the members' needs must come first. When this situation arises, experienced group leaders may take time outside the group to share their thoughts and feelings about leading a group.

The learner can gain much by becoming involved in **discussions** about the planning and evaluation of a group. If a learner joins in the planning process prior to a group, he or she will be exposed to all the decisions, considerations and preparations a leader makes. After the group session, learners can observe, at first hand, the processes of recording, reporting and evaluation.

EXPERIENTIAL TRAINING

An essential precursor to running any group is to be a group member oneself. Experiencing a group helps us to make sense of theory and enhances our self knowledge. Moreover, we have a professional responsibility to understand the experience of being in a group, before imposing it on others. This section explores these reasons why we should experience groups and then offers suggestions for where to go for experiential training.

The value of experiential training

Having experience as a group member helps us to **make sense of theory** and deepens our awareness of group processes. We need to do more than understand group concepts at a 'head level', we need to feel them – to know what it is like to be threatened by a group, to be scapegoated, to be excluded from a clique or to have unrealistic expectations of a leader. Exploring our own struggles in a group develops our capacity to understand and to empathize with our future group members.

Howe and Schwartzberg (1986, p 239) advocate that all student groupworkers should experience a group. They describe the benefits of this as follows.

> Only through direct experience can the student realize the power of a group and see how this power can be used to promote healing or cause trauma and pain. Through personal experience, the student develops an awareness of the importance of group acceptance, the difficulty of revealing feelings, especially positive feelings and the courage necessary to test reality and change specific ways of behaving.

Being part of an experiential group can also **enhance our self knowledge** if we are open to it. We can gain insight into our behaviour in groups and self awareness of how we relate to others. Through group members' feedback we can better understand how our behaviour impacts on others. Do we make others feel valued? Do we set people's backs up? Do others fall into patterns of reacting to us, such as being nurturing? Why? Our particular biases may hamper our receptivity. Through group experience we can examine our values and prejudices more closely and see if we impose them unconsciously onto others. In a sense, being in a group puts us at the receiving end of 'therapy' where we have the opportunity to explore our feelings, motivations, needs and, importantly, identify any 'unfinished business' that could distort our perceptions of others in the future.

Beyond growth and development, we also have an **ethical and professional responsibility** to put ourselves on the receiving end of groupwork. At the very least, we should try out group exercises on ourselves, in order to understand how they feel, before imposing them on our patients or clients. We need to have the courage to face a group experience before we expect it of others.

Training opportunities

So where do we go for experiential training? There are a multitude of training and self development opportunities. Here are a few ideas to follow up if you are interested.

Academic courses

Many higher education institutions offer a range of relevant diploma and degree courses. You might consider, for example, doing a MSc in Psychotherapy at your local university. (Done on a part-time basis, these are normally spread over 2 years.)

National Health Service courses

A number of short courses or seminars may come up in your district which could be useful (and possibly free!) The Department of Psychotherapy in your district or region is often a useful source to tap for both training seminars and staff supervision.

Local groups

Why not consider joining a local community group? The many societies and self-help groups available offer a range of group experiences and support. Some options to think about are: single parents groups; women's or men's groups; Alcoholics Anonymous; gay and lesbian societies; church groups.

Local courses

Innumerable relevant courses and workshops are available in most regions – in fact, the numbers seem to grow daily as more therapist-come-trainers seek to 'income generate'! The workshops may be expensive but intensive short groupwork can offer some powerful learning experiences. How about joining several weekend dramatherapy workshops or alternatively a certificated day-release course?

Institute of Group Analysis

This institute is well known and offers an introductory course and one which qualifies you as a group analyst as well as a range of special events and workshops. The additional in-depth training on psychodynamic approaches they offer can be a useful supplement to your basic training. The address for further information is: 1 Daleham Gardens, London NW3 5BY.

Association of Therapeutic Communities

This association provides training workshops and conferences, and produces a journal. Their focus is often on groupwork. The address for further information is: Peper Harrow Foundation, 14 Charter House Square, London, EC1 6AX.

Post-graduate training courses in Dramatherapy

The post-graduate diploma in Dramatherapy involves joining a 1 year full-time or 2 year part-time course. Currently, at the time of writing, there are five training courses in the United Kingdom: Hertfordshire College of Art and Design, St Albans; University College of Ripon and York St John, York; South

Devon Technical College, Torquay; Central School of Speech and Drama, London; The Institute of Dramatherapy, London (a 4 year part-time course). The Hertfordshire College of Art and Design also offers Art therapy and Dance Movement Therapy course and an MA in Art Therapy or Dramatherapy.

The Scottish Institute of Human Relations

This institute offers lectures, workshops and training programmes in psychoanalytical psychotherapy, family therapy and groupwork. They also offer a range of services including personal counselling and consultancy. The address for further information is: 56 Albany Street, Edinburgh, EH1 3QR or 21 Elmbank Street, Glasgow, G2 4PU.

In this chapter I have sought to stress the importance of continued support and guidance in the form of supervision and group experiences in order to develop our skills as a group leader. The process of learning is never easy. It can be painful and frustrating but it can also be exciting and satisfying – and even fun! Groupwork is always a challenge whether you are a group member or leader.

For all the highs and lows you will undoubtedly experience in your groups, I wish you a good journey.

Further reading

GROUPWORK THEORY

Cartwright, D.A. and Zander, A. (eds) (1968) *Group Dynamics Research and Theory*, 3rd edn, Tavistock Publications, London.

Corey, M.S. and Corey, G. (1987) *Groups: Process and Practice*, 3rd edn. Brooks/Cole Publishing Company, California.

Heap, K. (1977) *Group Theory for Social Workers: an Introduction*. Pergamon Press, Oxford.

Whittaker, D.S. (1985) *Using Groups to Help People*. Routledge and Kegan Paul, London.

Yalom, I.D. (1975) *The Theory and Practice of Group Psychotherapy*, 2nd edn. Basic Books, New York.

Bion, W.R. (1961) *Experiences in groups*, Tavistock publications, London.

OCCUPATIONAL THERAPY GROUPWORK

Borg, B. and Bruce, M.A. (1991) *The Group System: the Therapeutic Activity Group in Occupational Therapy*. Slack Incorporated, New Jersey.

Fidler, G.S. and Fidler, J.W. (1963) *Occupational Therapy: a Communication Process in Psychiatry*. The Macmillan Company, New York.

Gibson, D. (1988) *Group Process and Structure in Psychosocial Occupational Therapy*. The Haworth Press, New York.

Howe, M. and Schwartzberg, S. (1986) *A Functional Approach to Group Work in Occupational Therapy*. J.B. Lippincott, Philadelphia.

Kaplan, K.L. (1988) *Directive Group Therapy*. Slack Incorporated, Thorofare, New Jersey.

Mosey, A.C. (1973) *Activities Therapy*. Raven Press, New York.

GROUPWORK IDEAS

Brandes, D. and Phillips, H. (1979) *Gamesters Handbook.* Hutchinson, London.

Hutchins, S. Comins, J. and Offiler, J. (1991) *The Social Skills Handbook: Practical Activities for Social Communication.* Winslow Press, Oxford.

Jennings, S. (1986) *Creative Drama in Groupwork.* Winslow Press, Oxford.

Liebmann, M. (1986) *Art Therapy for Groups: a Handbook of Themes, Games and Exercises.* Croom Helm, London.

Napier, R. and Gershenfeld, M. (1983) *Making Groups Work: a Guide for Group Leaders.* Houghton Miffin Company, Boston.

Remocker, J. and Storch, E. (1982) *Action Speaks Louder: Handbook of Non-verbal Group Techniques.* Churchill Livingstone, Edinburgh.

References

Allen, C. (1985) *Occupational Therapy for Psychiatric Diseases: Measurement and Management of Cognitive Disabilities.* Little, Brown and Co., Boston.

Applbaum, R.L., Anatol, K., Hays, E.R. *et al.* (1973) *Fundamental Concepts in Human Communication.* Cranfield Press, New York.

Argyle, M. (1967) *The Psychology of Interpersonal Behaviour.* Penguin, London.

Argyle, M. (1987) Some new developments in social skills training. In *Language, Communication and Education,* (eds B.M. Mayor and A.K. Pugh). Croom Helm, London.

Axline, V.M. (1989) *Playtherapy.* Churchill Livingstone, Edinburgh.

Azima, H., and Azima F. (1959) Projective group therapy. *International Journal of Group Psychotherapy,* **9**, 176–83.

Azima, H., Cramer-Azima, F. and Wittkower, E.G. (1957). Analytic group art therapy. *International Journal of Group Psychotherapy,* **7**, 243–60.

Bales, R.F. (1970) *Personality and Interpersonal Behaviour.* Holt, Rhinehart and Winston, New York.

Bavelas, A. (1950) Communication patterns in task-oriented groups. In *Group Dynamics Research and Theory,* 3rd edn, (eds D.A. Cartwright and A. Zander) Tavistock Publications, London, pp 503–11.

Benne, K.D. and Sheats, P. (1948) Functional roles of group members, *Journal of Social Issues,* **4**, 41–9.

Benson, J.F. (1987) *Working more Creatively with Groups.* Tavistock Publications, London.

Blair, S.E.E. (1979) Supportive psychotherapy groups with the elderly, *British Journal of Occupational Therapy,* **June 1979**, 137–8.

Index

Blair, S. (1990) Occupational therapy and group psychotherapy. In *Occupational Therapy in Mental Health*, (ed. J. Creek), Churchill Livingstone, Edinburgh, pp 193–210.

Brady, J.P. (1984) Social skills training for psychiatric patients, I: concepts, methods and clinical results. *Occupational Therapy and Mental Health*, **4**, 51.

Clark, E. and Keeble, S. (1987) *Communication and Group Behaviour*. Distance Learning Centre, South Bank Polytechnic, London.

Clark, J.B. and Culbert, S.A. (1965) Mutually therapeutic perception and self-awareness in a T-group, *Journal of Applied and Behavioural Science*, **1**, 180–94.

De-Carlo, J.J. and Mann, W.C. (1985) The effectiveness of verbal versus activity groups in improving self perceptions of interpersonal communication skills, *American Journal of Occupational Therapy*, **39(1)**, 20–7.

De Mare P.B. and Kreegar, L.C. (1974) *Introduction to Group Treatments in Psychiatry*. Butterworth, London.

Dickoff, H. and Lakin, M. (1963) Patients' views of group psychotherapy, *International Journal of Group Psychotherapy*, **13**, 61–73.

Duncombe, L.W. and Howe, M.C. (1985) Groupwork in occupational therapy: a survey of practice. *American Journal of Occupational Therapy*, **39(3)**, 163–70.

Earhart, C. (1985) Occupational therapy groups. In *Occupational Therapy for Psychiatric Diseases: Measurement and Management of Cognitive Disabilities* (ed. C. Allen), Little, Brown and Co., Boston.

Festinger, L. (1954) A theory of social comparison processes. *Human Relations*, **7(2)**, 117–40.

Fidler, G.S. and Fidler, J.W. (1963) *Occupational Therapy: a Communication Process in Psychiatry*. The Macmillan Company, New York.

Fiedler, F.E. (1968) Personality and situational determinants of leadership effectiveness. In *Group Dynamics Research and Theory*, 3rd edn (eds D.A. Cartwright and A. Zander), Tavistock Publications, London, pp 362–80.

Franklin, L. (1990) Social skills training. In *Occupational Therapy in Mental Health*, (ed. J. Creek), Churchill Livingstone, Edinburgh, pp 193–210.

Gough, H.G. (1957) *Manual for the California Psychological*

Inventory. Consulting Psychologists' Press, Palo Alto, California.

Haley, J. (1976) *Problem Solving Therapy*. Jossey Bass, San Francisco.

Hargie, O., Saunders, C. and Dickson, D. (1981) *Social Skills in Interpersonal Communication*. Croom Helm, London.

Heap, K. (1977) *Group Theory for Social Workers: an Introduction*. Pergamon Press, Oxford.

Heinicke, C. and Bales, R.F. (1953) Development trends in the structure of small groups, *Sociometry*, **16**, 7–39.

Henry, A., Nelson, D. and Duncombe, L. (1984) Choice making in group and individual activity. *American Journal of Occupational Therapy*, **38**, 245–325.

Howe, M. and Schwartzberg, S. (1986) *A Functional Approach to Group Work in Occupational Therapy*. J.B. Lippincott, Philadelphia.

Janis, I.L. (1972) *Victims of Group Think: a Psychological Study of Foreign Policy Decisions and Fiascos*. Houghton Mifflin, Boston, Mass.

Kanas, N. (1986) Group therapy with schizophrenics: a review of controlled studies. *International Journal of Group Psychotherapy*, **36**, 339–51.

Kaplan, K.L. (1988) *Directive Group Therapy*. Slack Incorporated, Thorofare, New Jersey.

Kielhofner, G. (ed.) (1985) *A Model of Human Occupation: Theory and Application*. Williams and Wilkins, Baltimore.

Klyczek, J. and Mann, W. (1986) Therapeutic modality comparisons in day treatment. *American Journal of Occupational Therapy*, **40**, 606–11.

Kremer, E.R.H., Nelson, D. and Duncombe, L. (1984) Effects of selected activities on affective meaning in psychiatric patients. *American Journal of Occupational Therapy*, **38**:8, 522–8.

Lewin, K. (1948) *Resolving Social Conflicts: Selected Papers on Group Dynamics*. Harper, New York.

Lewin, K., Lippitt, R. and White, R. (1939) Patterns of aggressive behaviour in experimentally designed social climates, *Journal of Social Psychology*, **10**, 271–99.

McDermott, A. (1988) The effect of three group formats on group interaction patterns. In *Group Process and Structure in Psycho-Social Occupational Therapy*, (ed, D. Gibson), The Haworth Press, New York, pp 69–89.

Merton, R.K. (1957) *Social Theory and Social Structure*. Free Press, Glencoe, Illinois.

Monroe, C.J. and Herron, S. (1980) Projective art used as an integral part of an intensive group therapy experience. *British Journal of Occupational Therapy*, **January 1980**, 21–4.

Moreno, J.L. (1946) *Psychodrama*. Beacon House, New York.

Moreno, J.L. (1953) *Who shall survive?* (revised edition), Beacon House, New York.

Moscovici, S. and Zavalloni, M. (1969) The group as a polarizer of attitudes. *Journal of Personality and Social Psychology*, **12**, 125–35.

Mosey, A.C. (1973) *Activities Therapy*. Raven Press, New York.

Mosey, A.C. (1986) *Psychosocial Components of Occupational Therapy*. Raven Press, New York.

Nichols, K. and Jenkinson, J. (1991) *Leading a Support Group*. Chapman and Hall, London.

Perls, F. (1974) *The Gestalt Approach and Eye Witness to Therapy*. Science and Behaviour Books, Ben Lomond, California.

Priestley, P. and McGuire, J. (1983) *Learning to help: Basic Skills Exercises*. Tavistock Publications, New York.

Rogers, C.R. (1970) *Encounter Groups*. Penguin, Harmondsworth, Middlesex.

Schultz, W. (1958) *FIRO: a Three-Dimensional Theory of Interpersonal Behaviour*. Holt, Rinehart and Winston, New York.

Steinzor, B. (1950) The spatial factor in face to face discussion groups. *Journal of Abnormal Social Psychology*, **45**, 552–5.

Stewart, A. (1990) Research. In *Occupational Therapy and Mental Health: Principles, Skills and Practice*, (ed. J. Creek), Churchill Livingstone, Edinburgh.

Stoner, J.A.F. (1961) A comparison of individual and group decisions including risk. In *Social Psychology*, (ed. R. Brown), Free Press, New York.

Tuckman, B.W. (1965) Developmental sequences in small groups. *Psychological Bulletin*, **63**, 384–99.

Whittaker, D.S. (1985) *Using Groups to Help People*. Routledge and Kegan Paul, London.

Yalom, I.D. (1975) *The Theory and Practice of Group Psychotherapy*, 2nd edn. Basic Books, New York.

Yalom, I.D., Houts, P.S., Newell, G. and Rank, K.H. (1967) Preparation of patients for group therapy, *Archives of General Psychiatry*, **17**, 416–27.